Chronic
HOPE

Advance Praise

"In *Chronic Hope*, Bonnie O'Neil describes with firsthand experience how parents' natural desires for their children to lead happy and fulfilling lives can be challenged in myriad ways by a chronic disease. This book is enlightening and ultimately a source of reassurance for parents of children with newly diagnosed conditions as well as anyone who wants to understand their experiences and perspectives."

—**Derek Rapp**, former CEO of JDRF (Juvenile Diabetes Research Foundation)

"Type 1 diabetes requires around-the-clock care, with life and death decisions being made daily. Caregivers of children living with any chronic disease have a unique burden, taking an emotional toll for which there has never been a clear guide. *Chronic Hope* is that guide. Bonnie's experiences, advice, and insight form an invaluable resource for parents of the recently diagnosed, as well as seasoned caregivers experiencing burnout."

—**Thom Scher**, CEO of Beyond Type 1

"Before she was even born, type 1 diabetes was impacting author Bonnie O'Neil's life. In her new book, *Chronic Hope*, she takes the reader on a journey from devastation to renewal, providing validation and relief to any family living with chronic illness. Real and raw, her words draw you in and bring a sense of comfort, encouragement, and belonging. The "Heart to Heart" section at the end of each chapter affords the reader an opportunity to reflect on their own unique journey and offers the practical solutions families crave. *Chronic Hope* is an authentic guidebook for navigating the choppy waters of chronic illness—a lifeline that will pull you from despair ultimately to hope."

—**Sarah Lucas**, co-founder of Beyond Type 1

"When my family's life was turned upside down by the impact of type 1 diabetes, we searched for the playbook to tell us all we needed to know for our new reality. While we never found the book we wanted, we were lucky to meet Bonnie O'Neil and gained so much wisdom from her experience. Her new book, *Chronic Hope*, is a "must have" for every member of a family struck by a chronic disease. Bonnie packs the pages with the ups and downs—and at the end of the book, we are much wiser because of the experience she shares. Chronic Hope is a story of resilience, love, and unstoppable determination."

—**Matthew Cohn**, JDRF Global Mission Board member and Director Emeritus

"When a child is diagnosed with chronic disease, parents experience a range of emotions and the entire family dynamic changes. Bonnie O'Neil's personal anecdotes illustrate this myriad of feelings, so the reader feels validated and not so alone. Bonnie's wisdom and insight are profound and cannot fail to touch the reader's heart. Each chapter of *Chronic Hope* opens with an inspirational quote and ends with thoughtful questions that serve as tools to help the reader examine and process their own feelings. From grief to newfound hope, the reader feels like Bonnie has walked in the same shoes and shared their journey, which offers the reader peace and comfort, and ultimately, hope."

—**Elizabeth Weiser Caswell**, JDRF International Board, Vice Chair of Research

"I want to put Bonnie O'Neil's book into the hands of every parent I know, whether they parent children with chronic illness or not. *Chronic Hope* is beautifully written and weighty with hard-earned wisdom. Deeply personal and widely relevant, it will be most treasured by parents devastated by a child's diagnosis, parents worn out by worry or caregiving, and parents who can't seem to shake their fear and guilt. Bonnie stumbled along that difficult path only to find herself steadied by the persistent presence of hope. Her story will be a lifeline for many."

—**Christie Purifoy**, author of *Roots and Sky* and *Placemaker*

"Bonnie O'Neil's *Chronic Hope* is a brave and generous gift to every parent who has borne the responsibility of raising and caring for a child who suffers from a chronic illness. Speaking to us in a voice tempered by hard experience, Bonnie recalls the days and nights of watching and worrying, nights often made sleepless by the duties of care.

Chronic Hope is the story of a journey, tracing an arc that begins in desperation and reaches toward wholeness, toward deep insight, toward the hope of the book's title. This is an important and beautifully written book, honest, humane, and passionate."

—**Peter Conn**, author and Vartan Gregorian Professor of English Emeritus and professor of education at University of Pennsylvania

"Parents with a child whose chronic illness requires constant monitoring and treatment, brings on recurrent crises, and upends family life will find direction and solace in Bonnie O'Neil's reflections on raising a son with type 1 diabetes. Each chapter recounts a learning moment in the journey of caring for and equipping her son to take over his own arduous treatment. With emotional honesty and the authority of long experience, Bonnie offers parents hard-won hope. Readers whose lives haven't been touched by chronic disease will find their compassion deepened for those who live with illness as a daily, demanding fact of life."

—**Marilyn McEntyre**, author of *Caring for Words in a Culture of Lies* and *Speaking Peace in a Climate of Conflict*

Chronic
HOPE

Raising a Child with Chronic Illness
with Grace, Courage, and Love

Bonnie O'Neil

NEW YORK

LONDON • NASHVILLE • MELBOURNE • VANCOUVER

Chronic Hope

Raising a Child with Chronic Illness with Grace, Courage and Love

Published in New York, New York, by Morgan James Publishing. Morgan James is a trademark of Morgan James, LLC. www.MorganJamesPublishing.com

ISBN 9781631952289 paperback
ISBN 9781631952296 eBook
Library of Congress Control Number: 2020938861

Cover Design by:

Christopher Kirk, GFSstudio.com

Interior Design by:

Melissa Farr, melissa@backporchcreative.com

Author Photo by:

Brenda Carpenter Photography

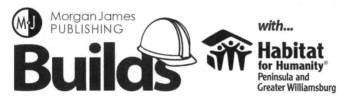

Morgan James is a proud partner of Habitat for Humanity Peninsula and Greater Williamsburg. Partners in building since 2006.

Get involved today! Visit
MorganJamesPublishing.com/giving-back

For Austin,
for always trusting me
and embracing life with courage

Table of Contents

Foreword

Raising a child with any chronic illness is hard. Raising a child with type 1 diabetes is particularly complicated because of the unpredictability of the disease and the need to provide round-the-clock vigilant care. Besides the countless tasks and rituals that must be performed on a daily basis, there are inconsistent short-term results and unpredictable long-term outcomes.

Having lived with type 1 diabetes for thirty-five years (and counting), and having managed and educated thousands of patients and their families for the past twenty-five, I can honestly say there is one thing that's more difficult than living with type 1 diabetes—parenting a child with type 1 diabetes. Why? In addition to the day-to-day challenges associated with managing glucose levels in a child, I see parents and caregivers dealing with an unsustainable level of *accountability*.

The glucose management part is difficult enough. Unlike adults, kids bring the complexity of diabetes care to an entirely different level. Very young children can be finicky eaters, have unpredictable levels of physical activity, and can be hyper-sensitive to the slightest changes in food intake and insulin dosing. School-age kids experience growth surges and ever-changing schedules which can lead to grazing rather than eating at predictable times. Teens and young adults experience surges in pubertal hormones, risk taking, and plenty of rebellious behavior. And that's all *in addition* to the usual variables influencing glucose levels.

The accountability part is unique to parents and caregivers. As an adult taking care of my own diabetes, if my blood sugar goes above or below where I like it to be, I can simply fix it and shrug it off. But parents have a natural tendency to feel responsible for anything and everything that happens to their child.

- *Glucose spiked really high after eating pizza? I must have undercounted the carbs.*

- *A low blood sugar in the middle of the night? I am making my child suffer needlessly.*

- *A1C went up by 0.5 percent? I have set up my child for a lifetime of poor health.*

The diagnosis of type 1 diabetes coupled with the inherent ups and downs of daily glucose management can lead parents into a cycle of guilt, frustration, and anxiety. And this, in turn, often contributes to poor decision-making and either insufficient or overbearing care for the child.

A healthy emotional approach to dealing with a child's diagnosis and ongoing management is the cornerstone of success. Too often, healthcare providers focus purely on the "numbers" and pay too little attention to what's going on in the minds of their patients and their caregivers. That's what drew me to Bonnie O'Neil's *Chronic Hope*. In it, you will find more than just facts and figures related to childhood diabetes. You'll find a sense of comfort. And peace. And balance. Whether you think you have it "all under control" or are desperate for answers, read it cover to cover. There are hidden gems throughout.

I first met Bonnie when she brought her son Austin to me for help in managing his diabetes, shortly after his diagnosis. We have known each other in this capacity and also as fellow board members of the founding chapter of JDRF—the Juvenile Diabetes Research Foundation—for over a decade. Whether managing her son's care or leading our local JDRF chapter, Bonnie is consistently passionate about and committed to improving the lives of those affected by type 1 diabetes. I think you'll discover in these pages a parent who has learned to lean into hope.

Remember, taking care of a child with diabetes, or any other chronic illness, isn't easy. Nobody expects perfect results. Heck, with most kids we're happy if they just show up. You've already shown up. Day after day, night after night. You show up regardless of all the frustrations and challenges and other responsibilities you have to deal with. And showing up is 90 percent of the battle. So give yourself a pat on the back! You deserve it.

Gary Scheiner MS, CDCES

Owner and Clinical Director, Integrated Diabetes Services LLC

2014 AADE Diabetes Educator of the Year

Author, *Think Like a Pancreas*

integrateddiabetes.com

Introduction

Shattered Hope

It's like in the great stories, Mr. Frodo. The ones that really mattered. Full of darkness and danger they were. And sometimes you didn't want to know the end...because how could the end be happy? How could the world go back to the way it was when so much bad had happened? But in the end, it's only a passing thing...this shadow. Even darkness must pass. A new day will come. And when the sun shines it will shine out the clearer.
— J.R.R. TOLKIEN

I press close to my five-year-old son, my hand stroking his tender back, tousling his blond hair. "It's just a game," I say when I ask him to pee into the clear plastic cup. "See if you can aim it all in there." Pleased with his success, he runs off smiling, returning to his enormous assortment of Legos to continue his latest building project.

My hands tremble as I remove the four-inch-long white plastic strip from the canister. Has my heart ever beat this fast before? It feels like it will pound right out of my chest.

I have used these strips many times in the past, throughout my childhood and during each of my three pregnancies. But never before did I feel like the world was about to shift underneath my feet.

1

I hesitate another moment before dipping the thin strip into the small cup of urine. *Will the result be unmistakably clear?* I wonder. Steeling myself against the result I most fear, I continue, lowering the white strip into the cup. The very second it touches my son's urine it turns deep crimson. There is no mistaking its meaning.

That was the day my heart shattered into a million fractured pieces, leaving behind jagged shards where once stood an intact, hope-filled life. June 17, 2002. The day my son was diagnosed with type 1 diabetes.

Chronic disease blew into my family like a cyclone, shattering our expectations of what should be and leaving in its wake the reality of busted hope. After the initial shock of diagnosis, we were left standing amidst the debris trying to gather into our hands the remnants of so many broken dreams. But like sand sifting through our fingers, those old hopes could no longer be contained. How could they be? They no longer held any substance. Overnight, they had lost their heft and slipped away, beyond our grasp.

In their place the stinging nettles of broken dreams took root. Fear became my constant and insidious companion. Desperate questions invaded my formerly calm thoughts. *Will I learn everything I must to keep my child safe and healthy? What happens during the night or when he's at school and I can't watch over him? What if I make an error in judgment and he doesn't survive my mistake? What is his hope for the future?* Fear gave way to anger as I struggled to come to a place of acceptance of our new life.

We may have received different diagnoses, you and I, but the nature of what we must process emotionally is remarkably similar. The day our children were diagnosed with a life-altering illness is a day we would never forget. Time stood still as our minds indelibly etched every fine detail of those twenty-four hours deep into our memories. Instinctively we knew we had reached the end of an era and would forever mark time by Before Diagnosis and After Diagnosis.

Perhaps you too have had a day that broke you. Or perhaps it was an accumulation of days and seasons and years that has left you heartbroken and exhausted from the responsibility of constant caregiving, and you too are overwhelmed from the fear that drives you to try to keep your child safe.

When disease imposes itself on a family, some days you feel like a prisoner to the disease, captive to the constraints of the disorder. You'll face seasons of heartbreak as you mourn what is no more.

When we embark on the wild adventure called *parenthood*, we bring with us our suitcases full of hopes and dreams for our children. We begin stuffing these bags full of grand plans before our first child is even born. We dream of holding our precious baby, counting all ten fingers, tickling all ten toes. Holding her until she falls asleep gently in our arms, nuzzling our face into the scent of her downy head.

We dream of endless games of catch with him in the backyard and teaching her how to ride a bike. We envision the goals he will score on the soccer field and the excellent grades she will earn at school. We dream of camping trips and sleepover parties, summer camp and a house full of our children's friends. We see their smiles, hear the laughter, breathe in the joy.

It is natural to hold high expectations for our children's futures, hoping they will enjoy lives that are healthier, more successful, happier—in a word, *better*—than our own lives. It is also to be expected that our hopes and dreams for our children don't include the possibility of them getting sick. And while we might not immediately articulate it as the highest dream we hold for our children, contained within every future image we have of them is that of a *healthy* young person. It is right, and good, for loving parents to hope for the best in life for their children, and it is equally fitting that we hope for them to enjoy good health.

Chronic disease never factors into our dreams for our families.

And yet chronic disease seeped into every pore of my family, as I'm sure it has seeped into yours. It has disrupted my marriage. It has complicated my relationship with my son, as I struggle with being his mother and caregiver without being a hoverer. The weight of disease has even affected my other children. Chronic illness is the great disrupter. Meals around the family table, dinners out, summer camp, vacations, the school day, the caregiver's day, a night out, a night of sleep—all disrupted. All shattered dreams. Days are no longer lived in carefree abandon; spontaneity has given way to deliberate planning.

While it is my son who *lives* with type 1 diabetes, the disease has also invaded *me* personally and has not left any single aspect of my life untouched or unaltered. Refusing to be ignored, it chiseled into the deepest parts of my being, forcing me to dig deeper for strength than I ever needed to before. An aching loneliness and alienation settled deep within my bones as I realized my closest friends were no longer able to completely understand my deepest longings and fears. Try as they might, it's nearly impossible to understand life with chronic disease unless you live it.

But you understand it because you're living it, or you wouldn't be holding this book in your hands. And I lived it, or I wouldn't have written this book.

So we meet on these pages—two caregivers who know sleepless nights and shattered dreams. No matter what illness your child has, we share common struggles, fears, questions, and feelings. We can describe the hum and buzz of hospital machines as we sit bedside. We share similarly crowded calendars, filled with medical appointments with specialists in more fields than we ever knew existed. We whisper similar fears and prayers for our child each night as we drift off to sleep.

And we wake every morning to a life defined by chronic disease.

The road ahead is not an easy one. If you've been on this journey any length of time, you already know that. The undoing of my captivity to fear and anger, mourning and brokenness, required the relinquishing of my constant longing to live a different life. An easier life. A life where loving and caregiving didn't hurt quite so much. This is my search for a way forward, out of the mire, paved in hope and love.

The undoing of my captivity to fear and anger, mourning and brokenness, required the relinquishing of my constant longing to live a different life.

I do not share these stories of my journey of hope in chronological order. Their shape is not linear but rather forms a spiral, like a spiral shell, beginning deep within the caregiver's heart. From there the stories circle outward to the caregiver's relationships with the child and other family members, and eventually out into the wider world. I long for you also to find your way forward and that together, in these pages, we will step into hope.

On the day of my son's diagnosis, I realized we had reached the end of the life I had known and loved. All I could envision was a future filled with constraints, worry, and sorrow. What I discovered instead was the beginning of a life filled with greater compassion, strength, and genuine love. What I discovered was a heart beating with chronic hope.

Prelude

Hope Disrupted

Hope is the driving power and outermost edge of faith.
Hope stands up to its knees in the past and keeps its eyes on the future.
— FREDERICK BUECHNER

My story with chronic illness actually begins before I was born. It was a slower time, a peaceful time. John F. Kennedy was in the White House, Americans dreamed of putting a man on the moon, and little boys pretended to be cowboys in the Wild West.

The young family is living in a tidy post-war house in suburban Philadelphia. The woman lets her body drop into the sofa and catches her breath as she gently places her swollen feet onto the ottoman. Heavily pregnant with her third child, the thirty-nine-year-old woman is understandably exhausted. Her six-year-old daughter, Barbara, has just recovered from an intestinal virus, and now her eight-year-old son, Johnnie, is enduring the same bouts of vomiting his sister experienced. This was not the Christmas week this expectant mother had anticipated.

This has lasted too long, she thinks. *He seems lethargic; he has slept too much today. Something isn't right.*

Willing her body to rise, she finds her way to the phone. After a quick call to the pediatrician, the couple bundles up their young son and takes him to the hospital. There would be no New Year's Eve merriment for them this year.

Words are exchanged, vitals taken. Blood is drawn, but there would be a delay in learning the results. It is a holiday weekend, after all, and the lab is closed. Doctors scramble. Off-duty personnel interrupt their New Year's Eve plans and report to duty. The doctor's suspicion is confirmed—the young boy is in diabetic ketoacidosis and has entered a diabetic coma.

This night, of all nights, is the night for making merry and dreaming of the future. This is the night for standing with friends and family to declare that, come what may, there is hope that the next 365 days will be good days, prosperous days, days of health and happiness and peace.

But not this year. Not for this couple. This year, their New Year's dreams would be replaced with fear, and hope would give way to despair.

The following three days are a blur of anxiety, filled with words the couple hardly comprehend and marked by the deepest sense of desperation they have ever known. They hear the doctor's words as if through a tunnel—*I'm sorry, there was nothing more we could do*—and their world would never be the same.

My parents return home from the hospital brokenhearted and empty-handed. Nine days later, they would return to the same hospital, this time emerging with a newborn baby girl, Betsy, and a heart torn between grief and their responsibility to love and nourish this new life.

How do two loving parents process the magnitude of losing one child and gaining another in the span of nine days?

How does a six-year-old girl comprehend the death of her only brother and transition from youngest child to only child to oldest child in the same nine-day span of time?

How we process loss matters. It matters deeply. We, every one of us, hold despair and hope in tension in every hardship we experience. Choosing despair is clearly the easier option. Despair's invitation is deep and wide as it swallows us into its embrace. Hope, on the other hand, remains ever the gentleman, waiting to receive an invitation from the one who has discovered a vision that transcends his own strength.

My parents chose hope. They chose courage. They chose love. Deciding to expose their hearts to the risk of further injury and loss, they made the courageous decision to have one more child, even though, by then, they were both in their forties.

Eighteen months after the death of my brother, I entered the world with the usual operatic cries accompanied by a ballet of flailing limbs. Quickly, I was swaddled in a bundle of soft blankets—and perhaps an extra measure of hope.

I was born on the shadow side of death, but I was raised in the light of faith and hope.

My birth family is older now as the calendar marks off eight more years since I was born. It is said time has its inevitable way of healing. I'm not sure that time actually healed anything, but at least it allowed us to move forward. Nearly ten years after my brother's death, there is still no talk of the one they lost—some memories are too painful to revisit.

The day begins like any other. I leave home, spend the next six-and-a-half hours happily at school, and then make the return trip home by big yellow school bus. Barreling down the bus steps, it's a quick dash across my front lawn and up the single cement step to fling open the front door of the house that for nearly twenty years has borne witness to our stories of life and death, joy and sorrow, hope and despair.

Dropping my belongings as I make my way to the kitchen, I see her standing there alone. She is beautiful even then, with eyes pooling like saucers to catch the overflow from her sad eyes. There are moments when you know the wind is about to shift. The quiet before the storm when the world freezes and you take in every fine detail of the moment. I suddenly remember the details I had almost overlooked—Barb's bedroom was dark when I pushed open the front door, and there was no sound coming from the den TV or anywhere else in the house. Why wasn't she home from school?

"Where's Barb?" I barely whisper the words.

"She's in the hospital." My mother swallows hard before continuing. "She has diabetes."

I gasp at the sound of the word. Diabetes means Death in my family. Is my sister going to die? Will I lose my sister just like she lost her brother? Will my parents return home in three days' time, empty-handed and brokenhearted yet again?

My mother reads some of the questions tumbling around my young mind and pulls me in close. "She will be fine," she weakly attempts to reassure me. "She will be home in a few days; try not to worry."

But I do worry. I worry because this word, *diabetes*, has reemerged in the language of my family. I worry that each of us siblings will in turn fall victim to this disease. I worry that it might be contagious, and so I keep my distance from my sister once she returns from the hospital. I don't want to get too close. I don't want to be next.

We discover in those places where hope has dried up, fear moves in to fill the void.

As difficult as it is to adjust to life with the specter of disease and death looming ever-present, we make every attempt to find a new normal. But we discover in those places where hope has dried up, fear moves in to fill the void. The fear that Betsy or I will get this disease is never far from any of our minds. My mother makes sure we know the telltale signs of diabetes—frequent urination and intense thirst. And so we watch, and we wait, and we hold our breath, hoping against hope that we will be okay.

PART ONE

Diagnosis

Chapter One

And Now There Are Three

Hope is definitely not the same thing as optimism.
Hope is an orientation of the spirit, an orientation of the heart;
it transcends the world that is immediately experienced,
and is anchored somewhere beyond its horizons.
—VACLAV HAVEL

Three decades pass and the disease remains underground, stealthy and silent, waiting an opportune moment. I have a family of my own by now, and I share my concerns about this disease with each of my pediatricians. I learn it's useless to test for type 1 diabetes (T1D) at every appointment; the onset of this disease is generally rapid and unpredictable.

"You know the signs," one of my pediatricians had assured me. "Just keep watch and you'll know if there's a problem."

And so once again I watch, and I wait, and I fool myself into believing that awareness and clean living are any kind of protection against the force of such a mighty illness. I hold my breath, this time hoping against hope that *my children* will be okay.

The final grains of sand pass through the belly of the hourglass, marking that the time has come. The warning signs appear almost overnight, and deep in my bones I know diabetes has reemerged in the warp and weft of

13

my family. These first moments of realization feel almost sacred, a private intimacy between mother and son, and I am not yet willing to invite a doctor into this space.

I move as if by instinct, without really thinking, and drive to my local pharmacy. There, I purchase a urine test kit, as I have used myself so many times, to test my son's urine in the privacy of our own home. This disease is deeply personal to me. If there is a diagnosis to be made, it is mine to make.

The hands on the mantel clock barely move as I await the hour to collect Austin from his preschool's day camp. Yet once I have him safely home with me, I find I cannot bring myself to ask him to come for the urine test. *Will he be worried? What if I don't know how to interpret the results? Am I just overreacting?* The soundtrack of my stalling plays over and over in my mind.

The hour hand makes its way a little farther along the dial, and I know I can delay no longer. I decide to make it into a game. Calling Austin down from the playroom, I assure him it will only take a minute.

His eyes twinkle, oh how they twinkle, as he runs down the hall toward me. Always in a hurry, this one.

Once again I long for Time to stand still, but like Austin, even Time is in a hurry today. Only my hand lingers, over the soft blond waves that frame his face.

He fills the cup. I dip the strip. And just like that the test is done. And just like that my heart shatters. Test strips don't lie—my five-year-old son, Austin, has type 1 diabetes.

Clutching the strip, sickened at the sight of its crimson color, I enter a spinning tunnel. The ground underneath my feet may still be solid, but everything around me is turning at a dizzying pace. Somehow I make my way to the pediatrician's office to confirm the diagnosis. The disorientation overwhelms me. I just want the swirling to stop. I can't imagine how I will ever make my way forward, and yet I know I can't turn back the sands of time.

Your diagnosis story is uniquely your own. Most likely, you didn't diagnose your child in your first-floor powder room. Chances are your trusted doctor told you, or it was an unknown specialist at a sterile hospital who broke the news to you. Perhaps the diagnosis came when your child was still in utero. Or perhaps it was during your child's adolescence. Or maybe, like me, your diagnosis story interrupted a life of Legos and fairy tales.

Whenever and however it happened, your diagnosis story contains elements of the sacred as well. The events unfold in an otherworldly reverence. We gather these deeply private moments in the life of our family and hold them close, protecting their memory. We understand that a metamorphosis has begun, even if all we can envision in that season is the death of a dream.

> *We are all certain of the same thing—*
> *life will never be the same.*

We are all certain of the same thing—life will never be the same.

Whether you knew much or nothing at all about your child's disorder prior to the diagnosis, in those early days it's easy to get swallowed up in despair. I know I did. Questions assault us from every side as we seek information on how to care for our child and try to understand how and why this could have happened.

In these early days when hope is elusive and despair is easily found, our greatest accomplishment is simply to keep going. To rise each morning and put one foot in front of the other, even if we have no sense of where we are headed or how we will get there.

We carry on because we must.

I learned a simple yet heavy truth as a very young child—had my brother not died, I would never have been born. Something inside me cracks in those early days post-diagnosis, and every question of justice and fairness that I have suppressed most of my life comes tumbling out. In desperate times, questions rear up much faster than answers.

How can it possibly be fair that the same illness would strike three times in one family? How can my parents bear the constant reminder of the son they lost with each new diagnosis of the same disease? Is it fair that, at least for now, I can keep my son while my mother lost hers so suddenly?

The questions turn even more existential. Why was I given life only to have this dreadful disease pass to the next generation through me? Why did my brother have to die so that I could live? Is my life really worth more than his? And what if it's not? What if my life is found wanting? How do I live so my life is somehow greater than, or at least equal in value to, what his life could have become?

Today disease is the victor and despair is its spoils. Where is the justice? Does any of this even make sense? My light has gone out, and without the light I cannot see hope waiting in the shadows.

Heart to Heart

- *How did you respond when your child was diagnosed? Did you, like me, feel like you were hurled into a spinning tunnel or that the ground had shifted underneath you?*

- *How have feelings about the "unfairness" of the diagnosis affected you?*

- *What questions do you continue to ask, even though you find no answers for them?*

Chapter Two

The Waiting Place

*No understanding of hope can be honest unless it reckons
with the absence of hope, the dark night of the soul
when nothing comforts and nothing reassures.*
—SCOTT RUSSELL SANDERS

We journey home from that first visit to the endocrinologist, stopping
at the pharmacy on our way. I don't know it yet, but my visits to the
pharmacy will one day outpace my weekly visits to the grocery store. It
is warm in our hilltop house that has no central air conditioning. The
moving company arrives tomorrow to begin packing up all the contents
of our Connecticut home for next week's move to Pennsylvania. *This can't
all be happening at the same time.*

And yet it is.

It must be eighty-five degrees in the house. Too hot to think straight,
I switch on the window unit and head straight to the refrigerator. *You
have to keep the unopened insulin cool, ma'am* rings in my ears over the
hum of the air conditioner. Without thinking, I open the butter and
eggs compartment on the refrigerator door and gently place the life-
giving liquid inside. Instinctively, from memories locked deep within, I

place my son's insulin exactly where my sister has placed hers for the past thirty-one years.

Of all the senses, smell is the most closely related to memory, for it has the capacity to awaken even deep memories long tucked away and forgotten. From the very moment I draw up that first needle of insulin, everything comes flooding back. The acrid, medicinal smell that is at once the odor of disease and the aroma of life smacks me straight between the eyes. Oh, how I have always hated the smell of insulin. I will have to learn to be thankful for this smell, choosing to breathe in from its vapors the elixir of life and not the reminder of the threat of death.

Are these really my hands drawing up the insulin? Somehow I feel disconnected from them, like they are my sister's hands and I am watching her fill her own syringe with the potent lifesaving medicine.

No, these hands are my own, and the recipient of this first of thousands of shots is my little boy, not my adult sister.

How did we even get here? The month began with the usual celebrations that accompany the end of a school year, and the farewell gatherings that will send us off to our new home three-and-a-half hours away. Still, my giant-sized mama ears had been on alert for a few weeks now. Every day after lunch, when Alexander was still at school and Alicia was napping, I would hear the slam-bang of the toilet lid crashing down on the seat. Not once or twice. More like three times *an hour*.

My ears register the sounds that tell me his urination is too frequent, but my mind is not yet ready to process what that means. I push it down; I have to prepare for a house move, after all. I try to suppress the warning signs—frequent urination and intense thirst—but like a soldier trained to recognize danger, I cannot, and my heart begins to race with worry.

We had been in New Jersey that weekend for my mother's eightieth birthday celebration, and I had asked my sister to test Austin's blood sugar. She didn't have her blood testing glucometer, she told me, because she had tested before getting in the car. Stifling my disappointment, I told her not to worry; *I was just being overly cautious.* But when a friend told me the next day that she had given each of my kids a Sunny Delight to drink on that warm Sunday afternoon before our drive back to Connecticut, *but had given Austin two,* I stopped dead in my tracks.

Just like that. That's how we got to where we are today. It was as simple as hearing my new friend say *but I gave Austin two Sunny Delights.* The next day our world changed forever.

A desperate fear—an overwhelming despair—accompanies disease. It settles in and envelops us. One question haunts: *Will life ever be normal again?*

I'm stuck in the liminal space of no longer but not yet. I am no longer in the peaceful days that preceded diagnosis, nor am I yet in the place of understanding and accepting what is. I cower in the place of shattered hopes, destroyed dreams, and all-consuming fear. Do you know that place? It is the Waiting Place, where we await the assurance of new life where now there appears only the shadow of death. In the Waiting Place we remain locked in our grief, longing for a new normal to emerge. I long for this new normal, but I'm not yet able to grasp it or to envision its shape and dimension.

> *In the Waiting Place we remain locked in our grief,*
> *longing for a new normal to emerge.*

Like you, I had many hopes and dreams for my son. Didn't we both hope our children would enjoy good health and a carefree childhood? I imagine you also hoped for a few opportunities to get away with your spouse from time to time. What has become of our hopes for a peaceful and joy-filled family life? I didn't dream of my son's childhood being focused on food choices and medication doses. I didn't dream of all the stress or worry, did you? I never envisioned the heartache or limitations I now see before me. I had hoped that my son, my beloved son, would be spared so much pain in his young life.

Where hope is fractured, despair invades to fill the void. I had hoped, expected, to be the protector of my young son; instead I have just witnessed the shattering of his tender life. Everything I did to protect him up until this point was for naught. Now every dream he might have for his own future will have to pass through the filter of living safely with diabetes. What kind of life is that?

My sorrow assumes a different flavor; it's anger, I think, or perhaps self-pity. I'm not quite sure. So I push it down. I don't have time for anger or self-pity.

I move through those early days, packing boxes, guiding the movers, scheduling appointments with new physicians in Philadelphia, and trying to learn the intricacies of raising a child with T1D. It stuns me that everyone I see is smiling. How can anyone be smiling when my entire world has just caved in? How can their worlds continue to turn smoothly when mine has just fallen out of orbit? Doesn't anybody know? Doesn't anybody care? Whatever force has brought this disease upon my son must have interrupted the very cosmos itself.

I look everywhere for answers. I'm a Christian so I open my Bible, where I read these words, "We rejoice in our sufferings, knowing that suffering produces endurance, and endurance produces character, and character produces hope, and hope does not disappoint."[1] A sneer forms on my lips before I can stop it. Already the disbelief is settling in. Hope? Where is hope? What if the suffering breaks us at the knees? What if it breaks us at the knees so the challenge before us isn't endurance but

---

1 Romans 5:3-5.

simply getting out of bed in the morning? And if that's what becomes of my endurance, then what in heaven's name becomes of hope? Sure, maybe hope doesn't disappoint, but what if hope dries up?

The end of my hope is the beginning of my fear.

I struggle to make sense out of life. What was a given is now taken away. What was certain is now questionable. The end of my hope is the beginning of my fear. Some unseen enemy has paralyzed my will to carry on, and I just want to curl up in bed and wake up released from this nightmare. This diagnosis threatens to be my undoing.

And so I wait in the in-between, left alone with my own shock, fear, and inner despair, bereft of any hope for a way forward. Stuck, quite simply, in the dark and desperate Waiting Place.

We have settled into the new house in Pennsylvania. School is about to begin again, and with it will come a whole new set of challenges to ensure my son is safe at kindergarten. Fear for his safety overwhelms me.

A friend from Connecticut rings me to see how we're doing. Her daughter was diagnosed at age three with cystic fibrosis. *Cystic. Fibrosis.* I know enough of my friend's life in the trenches to envision their reality— myriad drugs and multiple daily sessions of vibrating vest therapy. My friend has it hard too. Harder, I'm sure, than we do. Suddenly, five to eight shots of insulin and just as many finger-stick blood tests per day seem a far lighter sentence than what my friend's daughter must endure. My friend has become the sage, and I hang on her every word as a lifeline to my future hope.

"For months I could barely think straight. The sorrow was overwhelming." Her words speak comfort to me because finally I have been given *permission* to feel what I feel.

"Some days I could barely breathe. But this unbearable shock won't last forever. Grief takes time to process. It took nine months before I adjusted. Give it time."

Nine months.

"Trust me, the day will come when you wake up and realize the sun is shining again. Be strong and keep the faith that our kids will be okay."

Nine months for the earth to spin on its axis once again. I needed to hear that.

I needed those words from my friend, whose daughter's life expectancy is only thirty-seven-and-a-half years. I needed to know that I wasn't crazy, that although I felt paralyzed and helpless and lacking in any real ability to move beyond this stuck place, things weren't always going to be this way.

I needed to know that in time I would be able to find my way forward.

I needed to know that the sun would come out again, even if I had to wait a little while longer.

Alexander Pope's oft-quoted words float into my mind. *Hope springs eternal.* Those three words pass my lips when I see the play on words for the first time. *Spring,* as in to appear suddenly. *Spring,* as in the season that follows winter. Has there been a double meaning hidden in this proverb all along? Must there be a winter of dying dreams before new life and new hope can spring forth? In nature, death precedes new life. A kernel of wheat must fall to the ground and die to be multiplied into many life-giving seeds. If hope really does spring eternal, perhaps this bleak winter season of dead hopes and dreams will culminate in a new hope.

Heart to Heart

- *In what ways has your shock over your child's diagnosis paralyzed you from moving forward?*

- *What hopes and dreams for your child do you now fear will never be realized?*

- *If you're feeling stuck in the Waiting Place, can you allow for a small measure of hope that a new way forward will come in time?*

Chapter Three

Anger

*Hope has two beautiful daughters. Their names are anger
and courage; anger at the way things are, and courage to see
that they do not remain the way they are.*
—St. Augustine

The last of the moving boxes is unpacked. I learned long ago as a "frequent
mover" that what doesn't get unpacked within those first two weeks will
never get unpacked. While my external surroundings are coming together
in an orderly fashion, inside I'm a stew pot ready to boil over.

Can I just say it? I hate moving. Where my childhood was anchored
in stability, my adult life has been punctuated by instability, the inevitable
consequence of moving every two to three years. I prayed this move to
Pennsylvania would be different from my last two moves—I even prayed
there would be no medical crisis. The diagnosis feels like a kick in my
gut. How could the disease that snuffed out my brother's life, afflicted my
sister since she was a teenager, and caught the rest of us in its grip of fear
strike my five-year-old son the very week of our move?

Like hot lava boiling underground before a volcanic explosion, the
anger inside me begins to bubble up in earnest. It starts deep in my gut

and forms a braid with anguish and fear. It flies past my broken heart and lodges like a bullet deep into my brain.

Anger is new for me. I am more likely to make bedfellows with sorrow or regret or self-pity, but not anger. Questions spew from my mouth like a prosecutor's interrogation. *Why this disease? Why now? Why this week, of all weeks?*

I feel powerless against the force of my anger. If I've entered the five stages of grief, then I jumped right over denial—there's no time for denial when you're the primary caregiver of a five-year-old who requires constant care and supervision to stay alive.

I settled right into anger.

Furious, I seek someone—anyone—to blame for my son's misfortune. Logic tells me someone must be to blame. Maybe it's God, or the Universe. Maybe it's some ancestor with a faulty gene. Maybe it's me.

I can't stop accusing myself of having failed in a mother's basic responsibility of keeping her child safe. It's my role as my son's mother not just to love and care for him, but to protect him, to keep him healthy and safe from harm. So I place some of the blame on my own shoulders.

I'm a God-believer, so I direct my sense of injustice at God too. How could he dump such a burden on my little boy? Why must a young, innocent child endure such hardship? I hurl a pile of accusations in his direction as well. *Where were you in all of this?*

I sneer at the Universe as I struggle to understand why everyone else's lives seem straightforward while mine has become so complicated. Their days dazzle with possibility while mine are now dark and foreboding. I want what I no longer have, and some days all I can do in response is stand alone, hands on hips, and shout fury at the Universe.

My heart is restless and brimming with anger.

But in public I keep my anger bottled inside. Just as a tightly sealed fizzy drink explodes once it's shaken, I fear I'll do the same. I'm the new girl in town, so I try to hold it all together. When I meet new people, I smile and pretend everything is fine in our little family of five. But inside I feel the pressure building ever stronger.

Anger is the primordial response we humans experience when someone we love, someone we are meant to protect, is hurting deeply. The greater the love, the greater the anger.

In our desperation to make sense of what we can't understand, we often seek out someone or something to blame. But blaming doesn't satisfy or make us feel any better because it doesn't get at the underlying issue. The real issue is not disappointment with self, with God, or with the Universe.

The real issue is our need for control.

Control is my need to influence and determine the outcomes of all situations affecting my life. Control is my attempt at ordering the world around me, and it is my insistence that life conform to my view of how things should be. My son's disease has interrupted the carefully ordered world I envisioned for my family. It has shattered my expectations. It has taken away my control.

> *Control is my attempt at ordering the world around me, and it is my insistence that life conform to my view of how things should be.*

And so anger rises up within me.

I want control. I imagine you want control too. In our culture, we all crave control. Even the most spontaneous among us live under the illusion that with the right amount of effort we can be masters of our own destiny. Then the unthinkable happens and the illusion shatters like broken glass in a fun-house mirror, and we see ourselves as we really are—partakers in the mystery of life, not controllers of it.

We try to do all the right things as a parent. We eat well and take our vitamins when we are pregnant. We feed our children good healthy food, give them their vitamins, ensure they get plenty of fresh air and exercise, and make sure they get adequate sleep. We shower them with love and storm heaven with prayers over them.

And still we can't protect them from every danger.

Worse than discovering we are no longer in control, we realize we never were.

We live our lives looking for certainty, looking to embrace control. The headline question in any crisis is "Why?" "Why him? Why this disease? Why now? Why us?" "Why" is the most subversive word to our presumed façade of control, for in it we discover that we have no ready answers. Opening Pandora's box to the question "Why?" unleashes all the unpredictability of uncertainty that we have kept under lock and key for as long as we can remember. To give voice to that question is to place into relief the reality that we have no answer.

The only way to true peace is through the crucible of releasing control.

We long for the solid ground of control, don't we? Yet increasingly we are asked to embrace the shifting footing of uncertainty. It's natural to yearn for the peace you once tasted. But we will discover together that the only way to true peace is through the crucible of releasing control. To take hold of hope we have to release our lock-fisted grasp on the way we insist things should be. The way things once were.

A new hope can only be birthed out of our willingness to set aside our anger and courageously accept things as they now are.

Heart to Heart

- *Were you angry when your child was diagnosed? How did anger manifest itself in you in the weeks and months following diagnosis?*

- *Where did you try to cast blame in those early days? On yourself? On others? On God? On the Universe?*

- *How do you think your need for control has added fuel to your anger? Could this desire for control be preventing you from accepting things as they now are?*

PART TWO

Just Me

Chapter Four

Safe

Hope is the power of being cheerful in circumstances
that we know to be desperate.
—G.K. CHESTERTON

My heart begins to race as my mind fills with fear. The pediatrician slips a piece of paper into my trembling hand. On it are written the name and address of an endocrinologist whom we are to see *the following day*. Not today, the day of my son's diagnosis, but the following day.

Didn't the doctor hear me as I recounted my family history with this disease? My brother didn't survive the diagnosis, and he's sending us home as if he had just diagnosed my son with the common cold?

No shot of insulin. No instructions. Just a name and address scratched on a piece of paper casually slipped across the desk.

"You caught this early; he doesn't even have ketones." The doctor's words ring like Greek in my ears. Should I know what ketones are and how to watch for them? How can I keep him safe tonight if I don't even know what ketones—the apparent mark of danger—are?

This is all highly unusual. I know enough to know that children diagnosed with T1D are admitted to the hospital to be watched, to receive insulin, and for mom and dad to learn how to manage this new disease.

I gather Austin into bed with me that night; my husband is in Florida on business. I pass my first of hundreds, thousands of sleepless nights where sleep will be more elusive than a rainstorm in the middle of a drought.

The sun creeps through the slightly drawn curtains signaling it's time to face the new day and my new reality.

We see the doctor briefly before being whisked away by the nurse for Austin to receive his first of thousands of shots. She has me practice on an orange before she draws up a fresh syringe of insulin and pokes it into his tiny arm. My son accepts the shot bravely, but I can read in his eyes his belief that this is a cure-all shot, like the one-and-done vaccinations he has received.

He isn't yet aware that the earth has shifted underneath his feet.

He has had enough. He is restless to go home. How do I communicate to him that his new normal includes multiple daily injections of insulin? How will I keep him safe from overwhelming fear once he realizes the truth?

Back with the doctor, I discover a kind man, a man who also wants Austin to feel at ease. He ushers my son over to a treasure chest sitting on the floor in a corner of his office. It's stuffed with a selection of meaningless trinkets like children are sometimes offered at the dentist's office.

This is supposed to make my son feel better?

And yet somehow it does. It takes just a little of the sting out of what Austin has just experienced. I notice this, perhaps because all my senses are heightened in these earliest hours post diagnosis. Perhaps I notice because I'm desperately looking for anything that will ease my son's fears about what is happening to him.

A few days later, now living in Pennsylvania with the debris of moving boxes all around me, my mind seizes the memory of the treasure chest.

I realize if something as simple as picking a trinket from a treasure chest could soften the sting of the insulin needle piercing my son's flesh, then I certainly could create my own at-home trinket box. I rummage through the cardboard boxes filled with unpacked items, looking for something "treasure-worthy." Pretty, but not too elegant. More five-year-old bling than thirty-five-year-old fancy.

I spy the gold box, a gift to me from my son Alexander. By its shape it clearly held cigars in its former life, before the preschool teacher conceived plans to convert them into jewelry boxes for her students' moms one Mother's Day. Beads and buttons, pieces of discarded jewelry and shells adorn the lid. The entire piece was spray-painted gold. Lifting the clasp to open the box, my fingers stroke the piece of crimson velvet adhered to the bottom of the box.

Just the right degree of fancy for my five-year-old son.

I set to the task of filling it with grocery store and drugstore tchotchkes. All small things, nothing that would break the bank. Little capsules that dissolve when placed in a warm bath, revealing a hidden spongy dinosaur or farm animal inside. Colored pencils. Crazy erasers. Miniature plastic sea creatures and dinosaurs. Cheap trinkets that said "Don't be afraid, I've got you" to my son.

I ask him if he wants to go to the treasure box like he did at the doctor's office in Connecticut. Eyes widening with anticipation, he smiles a smile that lights up his face. He follows me to my bedroom where I present the little treasure box to him.

"Pick one," I say, as his hand riffles through the trinkets. "I'll leave the box right here, and you can come and select one after every shot," I explain to him. He runs off with his magic capsule, delighted to see what small sponge animal will emerge from within its cocoon.

The treasure box held more than just trinkets for me. It held the hope that I was alleviating some of my son's fears related to this new disease. I saw the simple pleasure he received with every trinket he selected from the box and knew that in time he would associate getting a shot with getting a treasure.

I didn't want him to fear the shots—they were what kept him alive. And I didn't want him to live in fear of the disease—he was too young to live in constant fear. I wanted him *to feel safe.*

I made the treasure box to tell my son, "You don't need to fear the shots. You don't need to fear the disease. I will protect you. I will stay one step ahead of this disease. I will keep you safe." But in those early days, my son was too young to understand much about T1D. He didn't like the shots, but he didn't fear for his future, nor did he even realize the risks involved if I got the insulin dosing wrong or missed a low blood sugar episode during the night. He just hated the shots.

I realize I'm far more afraid than my son is. I want my son to feel safe because *I* need to feel safe.

I want my son to feel safe because I need to feel safe.

If only there were a treasure box for us parents to dip into when fear rises up, trapping us in a mental loop of what-ifs.

My fears to keep my child safe began as soon as I realized my son had type 1 diabetes. I had lived with the reality that, despite her best efforts and all the love she had tucked in her heart, my mother hadn't been able to keep her son safe. Love and effort, it seems, are no match for mighty diseases like T1D.

Fear crept in that first day and established a stranglehold on my life. I lie awake during sleepless nights asking myself the same questions. Will he live? Will he die? Will I learn everything required of me to be his caregiver? How will I control his blood sugars when he gets sick? How will I recognize his need for a new insulin regimen as he grows?

With T1D in particular, extra burdens are placed on the caregiver to watch, observe, make decisions about insulin dosing, and draw up the insulin carefully and accurately. Not too little insulin—that would cause his blood sugar to rise too high, he would feel unwell, and it puts him at risk for complications down the road. And not too much—that could kill him.

I'm no doctor, and yet I'm expected to keep him safe amidst the complexity of this disease?

The stress of my new responsibilities overwhelms me. Some days my teeth actually hurt because I'm clenching my jaw so tightly. *Relax your mouth*, I remind myself. I redouble my efforts to understand everything about this disease as fast as possible. Furiously, I read and research, seeking knowledge as some talisman to protect my son from harm.

The reading is beneficial; truly, I must learn as much as I can about diabetes management. But it doesn't assuage my deep anxiety over my need to protect my son.

I know you've felt engulfed in fear as well. It comes with the territory of raising a child with chronic illness. But fear is not meant to be a dead-end where we remain captive throughout all our days raising this precious child. Our families need us to continue moving forward, despite the intermittent fear we may continue to experience.

As the emotional gatekeepers of our families, we must work through these new and painful emotions. Staying locked in fear teaches our children to be afraid. We can't live in constant fear for our children's safety and expect to instill in them the confidence that they are safe.

To move beyond fear we must accept what is. As long as we refuse to accept our new normal, fear will hold us in its grip. Acceptance allows us to face our fears, and once we face our fears, we can begin to deal with them.

> *As long as we refuse to accept our new normal,*
> *fear will hold us in its grip.*

In accepting this disease, I acknowledge my son's vulnerability and also my own.

I was never intended to carry the burden of guaranteeing my child's safety, and neither were you. No human being can fully protect his child against every bad situation. Yes, it's our responsibility to learn, read, think, and make wise decisions, but *all the outcomes affecting our children don't depend on us.* We are not the givers of life. We are to be channels not for fear but through which love flows.

My love for my child caused me to fear greatly for his safety. But what if there's a purer expression of love? Not a love that ends in fear, but a love that pushes through fear and vulnerability and points us to hope where we once saw nothing but dead-ends. Might this be the greater gift of love? Learning to love in a way that releases fear doesn't happen overnight. It's a process, so we have to give it time.

The trinkets in my treasure box were meant to say, "I'll protect you. I'll keep you safe. You have nothing to fear." I thought that was my son's greatest need because it was my greatest desire to protect him. It turns out the trinkets actually said, "I love you. I can't take this disease away, but I'll walk the road with you, always trying to ease your fear and pain."

In the early days my son took a treasure from the box with every shot, and occasionally an extra one for good measure on a particularly trying day. Over time, he began to skip visits to the treasure box in favor of dashing off more quickly to play. Eventually I realized I hadn't replenished my supply of goodies in a very long time. He had moved beyond his need for the treasures. He had received the most important treasure, my love and support.

Heart to Heart

- *In what ways has fear for your child's safety held you locked in its grip?*

- *What are some practical steps you might take to release fear? If you are feeling truly overwhelmed, would you consider seeking professional help?*

- *How do you model love to your child rather than fear?*

Chapter Five

Night

Only a life lived for others is a life worthwhile.
—Albert Einstein

I'm bone weary. The past several nights have required me to test my son's blood sugar frequently, and the sleep interruption is starting to take its toll. It's basketball season for Austin, now nine years old, so the extra exercise is causing his blood sugar to drop throughout the night. He has also been growing lately and that always causes spikes in his blood sugars. Between the growth spurt and the basketball, I have no idea how much insulin he really needs.

I look at my watch; it reads 10:30 p.m., one hour since I last tested Austin's blood sugar. I say a quick prayer that his numbers are in range and turn off the lights downstairs. Climbing the stairs, our dog, Reine, races ahead of me. She always joins me as I say goodnight to the children.

From the soft hallway light spilling into Austin's bedroom I locate his small hand from under the covers. Taking his left index finger in my hand, I pierce his tender flesh with the glucometer's lancing device. Pinching the tip of his index finger between my own thumb and index finger, the bead of blood forms quickly. I squeeze until there's just enough blood, and then I slip the strip underneath the red liquid. The meter begins its five-second countdown.

Five-four-three-two-one.

The meter registers a dangerous low of fifty-two. Suddenly wide-awake, I grab a Juicy Juice box from his bedside table. Puncturing the box with the straw, I slip the straw between his lips. Immediately he begins to suck until the box implodes, signaling all the blood-sugar-raising liquid is now in his body and not in the box.

Rummaging some more under the covers, I locate his insulin pump and pull it out. I need to turn down his insulin supply for a few hours. Pressing the necessary sequence of buttons, I reduce his insulin and place his pump back in the pouch strapped around his waist.

I'm thankful that through all this activity my son remains blissfully asleep.

It's time to contemplate my options. Go to bed, setting the alarm for twenty minutes, or stay awake as long as I can, testing my son in the same twenty-minute intervals. I don't have to think twice. I hate the feeling of confusion I have when jarred awake after twenty minutes of sleep. I head back downstairs, wrapping my robe tighter around me, forcing myself to stay awake a little while longer.

The dog is none too happy with this arrangement. Ever faithful, she gives a yawn and accompanies me back downstairs to sit vigil while I wait for my son's blood sugar to return to a safe level.

By midnight I can stay awake no longer. His blood sugar is still not where it needs to be, so I slip under the covers, this time setting my alarm for thirty minutes. In these dark hours when the alarm rings twice during each of my sleep cycles, I struggle to get to my feet, wrestling with the slumber that keeps me pinned to the bed. Once freed from the weight of the covers, I make my way down the hall to my son's room, trying to shake the confusion from my mind and willing myself to think clearly.

In the dark, by the light of my headlamp, I wait for the number on the glucometer, praying it will finally be over one hundred, allowing me to safely go off to sleep for the rest of the night.

Sixty-eight.

Oh, come on. He has consumed five juice boxes by now. Drink one more, sweet baby. I will be back again in twenty minutes to check on you.

I crawl back into bed, setting my alarm for twenty minutes, and close my heavy eyes. Eventually things begin moving in the right direction. I make one final test at 3 a.m., just to be safe.

It was a six-juice-box night. When the alarm rings at 6:30 a.m. signaling the start of a new day, I can barely lift my head off the pillow.

My eyes hurt as I try to open them. I can already feel how much my back aches—an indication of how little my body relaxed during the night. It feels like I've traveled on a jumbo jet through five time zones without sleeping when all I did was help my son make it through the night.

Jittery and unable to think clearly, I move as if in a fog. This is not the type of morning fatigue a slow cup of coffee will remedy.

As parents of a child with chronic illness, we're likely to experience chronic sleep deprivation. Whether we have to check on our children multiple times a night or they feel compelled to "check on us" throughout the night, our sleep patterns often suffer greatly.

My French friends have an expression for this type of sleepless night: *une nuit blanche.* A white night. It's the kind of night that never gets darkened by eyelids pressed tight. This is the kind of night that leaves you more exhausted at the break of dawn than you were when your body finally slid under the covers.

I long for a week of uninterrupted sleep. Even the early days with a newborn baby were nothing compared to this. When sleep interruptions carry with them elements of fear, they take an even greater toll on our bodies. *What if I don't wake up in time? What if his blood sugar drops too low and he has a seizure?* Our fears are real, and they propel us to get up when we would rather sleep. During the hours of the night watch, I dream of returning to life before chronic disease when I enjoyed sleep-filled nights and less stress-filled days.

During the hours of the night watch, I dream of returning to life before chronic disease when I enjoyed sleep-filled nights and less stress-filled days.

Your daily life is hard. It requires the physical and emotional stamina of a great athlete. The difference between the athlete and us is there's no prize awaiting us at the finish line. And for some of us, there is no finish line. Our prize is knowing we chose to offer steadfast and sacrificial love despite the myriad opportunities for fear and worry and fatigue to overwhelm us.

Genuine love always requires sacrifice. I used to think I understood sacrificial love—I'm a wife and mother of three children after all. Yet after my son's diagnosis I realized I had much to learn about loving until it really hurt. Raising a child with chronic illness requires us to make frequent sacrifices. We sacrifice our time, becoming full-time caregivers and learning all we can about the disease. We sometimes sacrifice our careers as we struggle to accomplish all that is required of us as caregivers. And all too often we sacrifice sleep as we sit vigil during the lonely nighttime hours.

To choose the way of sacrificial love is never easy. It's usually messy and often requires pain in the offering. The language of sacrificial love declares, "You before me."

Truthfully, I haven't fully accepted this disease. When I continue to fight his illness rather than work with it, resentment blocks me from loving sacrificially. Accepting how things are frees me to serve him with an open heart rather than a bitter heart. And wherever the heart is open, love can grow.

Some nights as I sit vigil, when fear is at its greatest and my sense of control is at its weakest, I remember my mother. I know she would have traded a million sleepless nights to have even one more day with her son. This vision jars my perspective and causes me to ask a new question. Is my heart open enough to fully embrace the parts of my life I cannot change so I might unreservedly love the child I hold before me?

As I learn to love my son well—by accepting life as it is and doing my best to care for him—real transformation can begin within me. When I demonstrate sacrificial love, I know hope is not dead. Where there is love there will always be hope.

Where there is love there will always be hope.

Likewise, I must offer myself grace when I most need it.

The day after a white night is especially challenging for us caregivers. Crushed by fatigue, our tempers are short, and we tend to overreact to people and situations. When I react out of sleep deprivation, guilt points a finger at me. *You're not doing a good enough job. You should do better.* The accusations are deafening. But if I can get still enough to quiet this voice, another voice emerges.

Be good to yourself. The words, barely audible, rose up out of my spirit one fatigue-drenched day after an especially difficult night. *Be good to yourself today.* Sometimes we need our inner voice to remind us that the nighttime work of caregiving is some of the most important work we will ever undertake. When we choose to sacrifice our own needs for the well-being of our child, we are choosing love.

Don't minimize this. The work you do is the greatest gift you can offer your child.

Being good to myself means redefining some of the expectations I may have for my day. I reevaluate my calendar, postponing appointments that can easily be rescheduled. I look for ways to say *no* to optional activities that take more of my energy and focus, and yes to activities that are in some measure restorative. I seek carpooling help from friends or fifteen minutes of quiet to catch my breath. Mostly, I offer myself grace to go slower than usual.

Accepting my own offer of grace creates the space I need to re-center.

Be good to yourself today is now my constant refrain. I hope you'll make it yours.

Heart to Heart

- *How do you experience the sleep deprivation and fatigue that often accompany raising a child with chronic illness?*

- *In what ways do you struggle loving your child and yourself when you are bone weary?*

- *What are some practical steps you could take to offer yourself grace and kindness after experiencing a white night?*

Chapter Six

Guilt

Into every empty corner, into all forgotten things and nooks,
Nature struggles to pour life, pouring life into the dead, life into life itself.
—HENRY BESTON

We're almost at my house when the conversation shifts to the day my brother died. I had driven to New Jersey to pick up my parents for a weekend visit. They were in their eighties and didn't drive long distances anymore. My mother sits next to me in the passenger seat while my father is seated in the back, absorbed in his daily newspaper.

"The doctor said the stomach virus set off a chemical reaction in his body that caused the diabetes to develop so suddenly."

I don't think that sounds exactly right; we've learned a lot about T1D since my brother was diagnosed. But I don't want to correct my mother. She rarely speaks about my brother's death, so I don't want to shut her down with a contrary remark.

"Maybe the disease had been brewing in his little body for a while," I offer.

"We never saw any signs of it," she responds quietly.

"If the disease had been quietly brewing, the virus probably triggered its acute onset," I respond. "At first he was vomiting from the virus, and then he was vomiting from the diabetic ketoacidosis. And you would have had no way of knowing vomiting was also a sign of DKA."

Softly, the words fall from her lips, "I gave him sugar tea to drink."

It all happened more than forty years before, yet she could remember it in vivid detail as though it were yesterday.

"I didn't know he had diabetes. I was giving him sugar tea to drink."

I'm pulling into the garage as my mother pronounces this guilty verdict over her life. My father, unable to hear our conversation in the front seat, begins the unloading process as soon as I put the car in park. A few minutes pass as we take their belongings into the house.

My mother moves slowly into the kitchen. I follow her there, allowing my father to take their bags to their room. Wanting to ease the weight of guilt she carries, my mind races to think of something to say to comfort her.

Drawing closer to her I ask, "Mom, how many cups of tea do you think you gave Johnnie that day?"

With the memory etched in her mind she replies, "Two, or maybe three."

"And how much sugar do you think you put in each cup of tea?" I venture.

"Just a teaspoon," she quietly adds, still not looking me in the eye.

"Mom," I begin, even more gently this time. "Do you know how many grams of carbohydrate are in a teaspoon of sugar?"

"No," she barely whispers, perhaps afraid of the answer.

"Four," I inform her. "Four grams of carbohydrate in a teaspoon of sugar. Mom," I say, taking her by the shoulders, "you didn't kill your son."

Looking up at me, her eyes are now filled with tears. Crying was not a luxury my stoic New England mother often allowed herself. As the tears spill down her cheeks, I am overcome with emotion for my dear mother, as I realize she has carried this guilt for most of her life.

As if the anxiety, fear, and fatigue of managing a child's chronic disease weren't enough, guilt sidles up to us demanding our attention as well. Perhaps you don't face it in the same way my mother did, but we all live with some measure of guilt.

As if the anxiety, fear, and fatigue of managing a child's chronic disease weren't enough, guilt sidles up to us demanding our attention as well.

Never a good science student, I nonetheless remember enough about DNA and genes from biology class to know that one's propensity toward disease is somehow coded in the genes passed across the generations. The inquisition begins. Why were our genes defective? Should I have had children at all, knowing how deep this disease runs in my family and that it's also in my husband's family? Was I wrong to want to have children?

Feelings of guilt begin to form.

The inquisitor takes another tack, going deeper still. Why didn't I recognize the signs earlier? Why couldn't I protect my child from this disease? What kind of a parent does that make me?

Guilt hovers like a low-lying cloud, heavy with pressure, demanding answers to unanswerable questions.

Even after years of managing my son's illness, I can still feel guilty when it seems I've failed despite my best efforts to do everything "right" for him.

Guilt is a prison. It causes us to wall-up emotions too fragile to be spoken, as if mere words were powerful enough to accuse us and send us to the executioner.

Guilt imprisons us with facts and lies that we repeat and twist into accusations against ourselves, and others, paving the way for shame and blame to fester and grow. Shame is a liar, coaxing us to accept a false version of the truth. Blame—whether directed at ourselves or others—gives us a place to direct our anger. Embracing guilt is not a healthy place for our minds to settle.

Where loss—of life, of dreams, of stability—shines a spotlight on the ready response of guilt and despair, hope stands in the shadows and whispers *there is another way forward*. To make room in our hearts for hope we must let go of guilt. A heart filled with guilt has no room to nurture hope.

> *To make room in our hearts for hope we must let go of guilt. A heart filled with guilt has no room to nurture hope.*

Freedom from the shackles of guilt begins with offering myself grace and forgiveness. As parents we often fall prey to the illusion that if we do everything *right*, we will succeed in protecting our children from all harm. This is a dangerous "if-then" philosophy to embrace, for it leaves us assuming far more power than we were ever meant to hold. The truth is we can't prevent every evil from touching our children's lives. We're just not that powerful.

When guilt threatens my peace of mind, I remind myself not everything is under my control. I offer myself grace, remembering I could not have prevented my son from getting this disease. I offer myself grace to make the best decisions I can for my son's care. And I try to forgive myself when I realize I will never get it all *right*.

The children fly through the back door, excited to see their grandparents after a long day at school.

I think about all that transpired between my mother and me that afternoon. I realize six little eyes are always watching me. They learn about life by watching me. The way I model self-love really does matter, because they learn from the behaviors I demonstrate to them. If I hold onto guilt, they will learn that shame and blame are normal and acceptable parts of adult life. If I practice accepting the things I can't control and offering myself grace and forgiveness in return, my children will learn grace is the best remedy for undeserved guilt.

My parents envelop each of their grandchildren in a warm embrace. I watch my mother as she hugs Austin. Is it my imagination, or did she hold him just a bit longer than she held the other two?

I gaze at her face. It looks softer, brighter than earlier today.

What was I seeing in her eyes? Was it peace? Was it joy?

Could it have been freedom?

Heart to Heart

- *In what ways has guilt affected you since your child's diagnosis?*

- *How do you process these feelings of guilt?*

- *What steps could you take to offer yourself grace and forgiveness as you release painful guilt?*

Chapter Seven

Alone

There is a friend who sticks closer than a brother.
—King Solomon

The lights dim as I settle myself deeper into the plush folding seat. I feel the coarse crushed velvet through my jeans and settle in for ninety minutes of silliness and laughter.

Not one for cartoons, I have to admit the idea of watching a feature-length animated movie is not my idea of a pleasant Saturday afternoon. But SpongeBob has always made me laugh, so maybe sitting through the entire *SpongeBob Movie* won't be so bad after all. Plus, I've seen the previews, and I'm curious to know how Baywatch's most famous lifeguard will be incorporated into a film about the crazy antics of a friendly sponge named Bob.

My fingers brush against the pile of the crushed velvet, rough one way, smooth the other. Rough and smooth, a fitting metaphor for how my life feels these days. Friends and strangers look at my family and all appears smooth and easy, like their lives, and yet here I sit, alone in a movie theatre. The lone adult guest among the group of fifteen children happily celebrating their friend's birthday.

I choose my seat carefully. Not too close—I'm not really an invited guest. The boy's mother and I are not close friends. Yet not too far away. There I loom, ever watchful, ever present, ready to provide emergency glucose if needed, ready to inject insulin when it's time for the inevitable pizza and cake that will wreak havoc on my son's blood sugars for the rest of the day.

This is how it is with every birthday party, every school field trip—I am always there, watching and waiting. And while I'm grateful I'm allowed to participate in all aspects of my child's life, this much togetherness feels uncomfortable. I feel in the way and very much alone. The French have a fitting expression for this type of awkwardness: *de trop*. It literally means to feel as though there is "too much" of you. That's how I feel on these days when I wish the floor would just swallow me up so no one would know I had even been there. There's too much of me. *De trop*.

It's a terrible thing to feel so alone in a crowded room.

Some days I manage my sorrow well. Other days my grief threatens to be my undoing. "He looks great," my friends declare, heads nodding to solicit my response that "Yes, yes, he's wonderful! Couldn't be healthier!" How can I disappoint them by shooting down their quick assumptions of my eight-year-old's obvious good health by painting a picture of our everyday routine behind closed doors? This is the reality they never see and never have to experience with their own children.

I long to tell them that his latest growth spurt has meant a complete recalculating of his insulin needs, which I determine mostly by trial and error during long, sleepless nights of glucose testing. I want to shake my head and correct them. He may look great on the outside, but inside my son struggles every day just to feel well.

Occasionally I do speak up, but most days I don't. Most days I nod my head in unison with theirs, smile gently, and quietly murmur, "He's doing okay."

It's human nature, after all, to attempt to brush past pain and focus instead on some hidden or perhaps imaginary blessing in the trial. The problem is I don't always want my friends to hunt for the silver lining. Sometimes I just want them to take off their shoes, cross their legs, and sit with me in the grief of all that was lost. I'm not talking about a steady diet of this, mind you; that wouldn't be helpful for me or for them. But sometimes I just need someone to be *willing* to listen to my fears for my son's future. *Willing* to catch my tears in their outstretched hands, tears for my broken dreams of an easier path for my son. Tears for the challenges he already endures and challenges he'll face for the rest of his life. Some days I just need someone to understand I will always carry a measure of sorrow, fatigue, and worry, and they won't break me by talking about it.

Some days I just need someone to understand I will always carry a measure of sorrow, fatigue, and worry, and they won't break me by talking about it.

But maybe I would break them. Maybe they can't handle it.

When family and friends are unwilling or unable to meet me in the pain, I feel abandoned and completely alone. But when they're willing to enter into the pain with me, I feel cherished and cared for. And comforted in knowing I'm not alone. Holding me in the pain is the most beautiful gift they could give me.

Like those who seek out the silver lining for its potential to bring me some measure of comfort, there are those who play the great equalizer, attempting to support me with the knowledge that every human being has his share of difficulties to deal with in life. And while I know this to be true, I also know *this* to be true—just because everyone experiences

pain doesn't mean everyone's experience with pain is the same. To pretend that everyone suffers to the same degree in life only cheapens what my son is experiencing.

What he has been called to is hard. And what I've been called to as his mother is also hard.

And so I convince myself *no one understands.* This mindset keeps me focused on what I don't have rather than acknowledging the blessings I do have. When I choose to put my life in the balance and weigh it against my perception of the ease and beauty of the lives I see around me, I open myself up to feelings of jealousy that always seem to lurk stealthily in the shadows. Some days there's a jealousy that rises up within me, ferocious and hungry like a lion. It's a longing for the carefree life I once had but can no longer embrace. It's a jealousy of anyone I perceive to have an easier life than I do.

I remember a fall day not long after my son's diagnosis. Driving by our local bakery, I spotted a young mother with her children in tow, stopping for a sweet treat after preschool. With regret I wondered why I never took the time for those impromptu visits when we were still able to eat sugary treats with ease. Through my windshield I glowered at the woman, whose life looked to be the antithesis of mine—undoubtedly picture perfect and full of ease. Her children must be healthy and smart and well behaved, and most of her dreams must have come true by age thirty-five.

And all this I concluded from the purchase of a couple of cupcakes.

All too frequently my heart cries out that everyone else has it so much better, so much easier, so much sweeter than I do. I fall for the lie that I am alone in this struggle. The aching hole in my heart cries out to be filled, and filled it will be, with a dangerous companion called *jealousy.*

Jealousy does nothing but isolate us further from the community of friends that tries its best to offer us support.

If I'm brutally honest, I have to confess that sometimes when I'm in this place of—let's call it by its true name—self-pity, I even sense that others are judging me. Maybe it's judgment. Maybe it's pity. Either way, it hurts and it isolates. I see it in the smug look of the one who tries to comprehend my pain but can't for the life of her fathom the depths of what I'm describing. There is a pitying smile from the one who looks at my life and concludes, *You must be doing something wrong to have merited all this misfortune.* A judging look asserts, *I am better, luckier, more favored than you, and my good life is proof of it.*

When your life is filled with chaos and medical disorder, it's all too easy to feel judged or pitied by those around you whose lives are relatively easy by comparison. Managing a chronic disease is exhausting work, and the combination of fatigue and sorrow can often leave us misinterpreting others and longing for what we imagine everyone else has.

The morning light falls softly in my bedroom, awakening me before the alarm rings. I lie there a while longer, not fully rested enough to get out of bed just yet. It was another long night of sleep interruptions and blood tests. I roll over and bury my face in my pillow. Just a few more minutes of lightness before stepping into the burdens of the new day.

How many sleepless nights have I experienced by now? Hundreds, for sure, as the years have advanced.

The first sips of hot coffee go down easy, warming me, comforting me from the inside out. My phone lights up with a text from Peggy, my first and best diabetes mom friend, the one who taught me more about this disease than any of our doctors have. She was up all night too—growth spurts in little boys with diabetes guarantee all-nighters for mom.

We commiserate, sharing a few choice words for this stinking disease, and wish each other a better day ahead. And as my phone goes dark, I realize I am not alone. Beginning with Peggy and extending throughout my local network of T1D parents, I have an entire army of friends who stand in the trenches with me every day, who live, sleep (or not!), eat, and breathe type 1 diabetes. We don't live in the same neighborhoods, and our children don't attend the same schools, but I have known them as long as I have known anything about my son's disease, and I know I can call on any one of them at any time.[2]

Together, we have received education about T1D, we have raised funds for research, and we have been mentored and served as mentors to newly diagnosed families. We have laughed together, cried together, and dreamed together of a cure for our loved ones. They are more than friends to me; they are family.

Sometimes I still struggle to remember that none of my friends can meet all my needs. In the same way that I must ask for grace and understanding from others when I require access to my son at birthday parties and field trips, so too must I extend grace and understanding to my family and friends when they don't give me the support I need. It's up to me to accept support in whatever way they can offer it and to forgive them for not being able to meet my every need.

The sun rises higher in the sky; soon it will be time to awaken my children for school. I can see things more clearly now. I see that I have expected too much from my family and friends who live in a world

---

2   My local community is the JDRF, formerly called the Juvenile Diabetes Research Foundation. With chapters located throughout the US and abroad, JDRF is an extensive community of people working together around the same cause. Their mission is to cure, prevent, and treat T1D. My online community is Beyond Type 1, where I find hope, encouragement, and practical advice for life in the trenches of T1D. Social media also provides many opportunities for connecting virtually with others experiencing the same chronic illness for support, ideas, and encouragement.

outside the sphere of my son's disease. How can I really expect them to understand what they have never experienced? If they haven't walked a mile in my moccasins, how can they truly know?

I give thanks for my friends in the T1D community. They are a precious gift to me, and because of them I know that even in my darkest fears and sorrows, I do not walk alone.

Heart to Heart

- *How have you experienced isolation as a caregiver?*

- *How do you respond when friends try to look for the silver lining when they ask about your child? How do you handle any feelings of jealousy over their healthy children?*

- *Who is your "tribe" you can count on to really understand your life in the trenches?*

Chapter Eight

Emptied

Love anything and your heart will be wrung and possibly broken.
If you want to make sure of keeping it intact you must give it to no one,
not even an animal. Wrap it carefully 'round with hobbies and little
luxuries; avoid all entanglements... To love is to be vulnerable.
—C.S. Lewis

We recently celebrated my son's seventeenth birthday. He has grown tall and lean, the picture of health were it not for the T1D. There's an early fall chill in the air when Austin comes home from school that day, dropping his backpack on the kitchen floor.

"I'm really tired. I'm going up to take a nap."

He had been a champion at napping as a young child, but it has been years since my son has taken a midday nap.

"Are you feeling okay?" I call after him as he disappears up the back stairs.

"Yeah, just really tired," he replies as he shuts his bedroom door behind him.

Two hours later, as if he had undergone a strange metamorphosis in the cocoon of his bedroom, the young man who emerges is visibly changed. He wears fatigue like a heavy cloak. A vacant stare replaces the usual twinkle in his eyes. The source of energy and laughter at our dinner table is startlingly quiet and withdrawn.

Back in bed by 9:30 that night, he is still exhausted the next morning when I try to awaken him for school.

"He must be fighting a virus," I tell myself, and agree to let him stay home and rest. As one day dissolves into two and then three, I grow increasingly concerned and take him to our pediatrician. She runs a few tests and sends us home. The following six weeks are a blur of more doctor's appointments, medical tests, and missed school days, as my once energetic and gregarious son grows increasingly fatigued, a mere shell of his former self.

Finally, we are sent to the diagnostic specialist at CHOP, the Children's Hospital of Philadelphia, who confirms the pediatrician's suspicions. Austin has POTS—Postural Orthostatic Tachycardia Syndrome, a disorder of the autonomic nervous system.

"The diagnosis is fairly straightforward," the specialist says, "once you know what to look for. Your son's heart rate more than doubles when he moves from lying down to standing up. Once pumped out of his heart, Austin's blood can't make its way against gravity back to his heart or his brain. Whenever he sits or stands, he's in a state of tachycardia."

I try desperately to process what the doctor is saying but find I have no capacity to grasp any of it.

"There are no quick fixes....We can try to treat some of his symptoms....Some kids get well, some don't...Fatigue and weakness are the hallmarks of this disorder....Some people end up in wheelchairs.... Deconditioning of the heart happens very quickly, so a strict exercise regimen is essential."

How can exercise be a crucial part of my son's healing when he can barely get out of bed in the morning?

The more I read in the following months, the more desperate and heartsick I become. The complexity and unpredictability of T1D have always frustrated me. Managing T1D now seems like child's play compared with the complexity of trying to control POTS. Even after settling into a regimen of seven different medications, partial school days, and attempts at getting frequent exercise, it's clear we're losing the battle against this ferocious illness.

The light has been extinguished from my son's eyes. I recognize the long, lanky frame of the one I love, but nothing in his face is familiar to me. Will my beloved son ever return to us?

My stress cup was already near the spilling-over point when POTS came roaring into our lives. At the time, my husband and two other children were each undergoing their own physical or emotional struggle, pushing them to the limits of what they could handle. I didn't have much capacity to absorb the blow POTS dealt me.

My son's condition lasted close to twenty months before he was fully healed. The darkest days were the first nine months. In desperation I promised to buy him a new Taylor guitar if he would go to the gym regularly. We devised a system of debits and credits to keep him accountable to his exercise regimen. Sure enough, like the doctor had said, the increase in exercise really did promote his healing. But eight months after his ordeal began, while in the early stages of improving health, Austin suffered a concussion while playing softball, and four weeks later, a broken wrist while playing basketball. Because the broken wrist didn't set properly, he underwent surgery three weeks later.

As I carried the weight of these new burdens, in addition to the management of T1D, I wrestled with this one question: *How much heartache must one family endure?* I know having a child with a chronic disease doesn't give our family a free pass from suffering other illnesses and life challenges. I know we're not exempt from trials just because my son has T1D. Yet I struggled with the seeming injustice of it all. When is enough *enough*?

When Austin was diagnosed with T1D, I was overcome with anger, which led me to abandon my faith. I drifted far from hope, lost in a sea of despair. Knocked over by a mighty wave, I could no longer find my footing. It took me years to rebuild my faith and years more to develop the habit of hunting for hope even in trying circumstances. I had come to accept that Austin's life would be hard.

But this kind of hard?

When Austin got POTS, I didn't dissolve into anger, nor did I experience another faith crisis. For that I'm grateful. But his prognosis was bleak. Mostly I experienced fear and sorrow. Fear returned stronger than ever, but it was different this time. I didn't fear for his day-to-day care or whether I would be able to act quickly enough in a crisis. I feared for his future. *What if the child I raised never returns to me? What if his eyes continue to be distant and vacant and he never finds a reason to laugh and smile again? What if he doesn't get well enough to live independently as an adult?*

Oddly, my fears for my son's future forced me to stay squarely planted in the present. This was neither an escapist response to avoid thinking about his future, nor was it choosing to put an overly positive spin on things, blindly assuming everything would be alright in the end. I didn't know what the future held for my son. All I had was today.

How do we stay tethered to hope amidst this kind of suffering in our lives? How do we make space for hope to grow when there's so much to fear and when crisis after crisis pounds at our door?

Because of my faith, my hope is anchored not in my own strength but in the God in whom I've placed my ultimate hope. Perhaps it's easier to stay connected to hope if you believe in God, but it's not impossible if you don't. Hope can always be found when we're ready to open our eyes to it.

*Hope can always be found when
we're ready to open our eyes to it.*

Even in my most despairing days, when I would open my heart just enough, I discovered seeds of hope all around me. I have seen hope come close in moments of love and tenderness shared within my family. A nod, a smile, an embrace are all promises of our love and devotion to one another even in the storms of life. My son's small acknowledgment of thanks for my care helped me hold onto the belief that all hope was not lost for his healing.

I looked for hope when I awoke my son for school on his delayed-start schedule and evaluated his condition based on what I found. If his fatigue was at a normal level, I carried on with the plan to send him to school. If he was unusually tired, I extended him grace and revised the day's plan. If he seemed at all improved, I stopped and gave thanks, savoring the glimmer of hope.

A friend sent a card. Her family had lit a candle and prayed for Austin. The sisters in their religious order would also be praying regularly for my son, she wrote. Another friend sent a prayer shawl that had been knitted specifically for Austin, as prayers for his healing kept time with the click-clack of the knitting needles. I imagined a circle of gray-haired women uttering prayers for my son as their needles would knit-one-purl-one, and it moved me to tears. I didn't fully understand these faith practices of prayer shawls and lighting candles, but I was swept away by the beauty of the offering. I gathered grace in my arms like a hungry peasant discovering a bounty of fresh food.

In the darkest of days, we must look up. Only when we look up will we see other hope hunters, and when we find them, we must surround ourselves with them.

Hope took on flesh in the person of my son's guidance counselor. When we were too tired to fight for accommodations, he fought for us. When teachers demanded too much of my son, his guidance counselor readjusted their expectations for him. As my son's junior year dissolved before our eyes and college preparedness seemed elusive at best, he assured us we would find a way forward.

In the darkest of days, we must look up. Only when we look up will we see other hope hunters, and when we find them, we must surround ourselves with them. They will hold us in our sorrow and point us to hope.

Heart to Heart

- *How have you responded when challenges other than your child's chronic illness impacted your family life?*

- *Take a few moments to think of some people who have offered you glimpses of hope along your journey. What did they do? How did their offering of love or kindness make you feel?*

- *How could a practice of hunting for hope help you in the dark days of suffering?*

Chapter Nine

Strong

*The world breaks everyone and afterward many
are strong at the broken places.*
—ERNEST HEMINGWAY

I wrote out my list of errands the night before. Today is a day to hit the ground running as I finish all the last-minute details signaling vacation begins tomorrow. Nestled in between stops at the dry cleaners and the pet supply store is a stop at the pharmacy to pick up my son's insulin. It's still midmorning, so I know I can get in and out quickly, without waiting in the usual late-afternoon lines.

"Austin O'Neil, O-'-N-E-I-L," I spell out for the cashier as she searches for my son's record on the computer. "It's insulin. It's in the refrigerator," I offer when I notice she hasn't moved from the computer.

"There seems to be a problem" is all she needs to say for my carefully orchestrated day to unravel before my eyes.

"Your insurance company has changed its formulary, and the insulin your son uses is no longer their preferred insulin. So it's no longer covered."

Does anyone care that it's my son's preferred insulin, I wonder?

My mind races to process her words. After a dozen years using the same insulin, we are, without warning, told he must use a different life-saving medication. This is his backup insulin in case his pump breaks, so I have to take a bottle with us on vacation. My choices are clear: purchase his usual insulin at full price, accept the new insulin—which he has never used before—or call the insurance company and plead our case.

I'm sure I snarled or growled at the cashier as I turned on my heels to find my way back to my car. Giving no thought to my remaining errands, I return home to call the insurance company. I explain our sad tale. "Yes, we're leaving tomorrow for two weeks overseas, and no, he has never used that insulin before." The agent confers first with a manager, next with the pharmacy.

They tell me I can request a pre-authorization from my son's doctor to receive coverage for the original insulin. We leave for vacation in twenty-four hours; there's no time to fight for a pre-authorization now. But maybe the pharmacy will work with me once I return from vacation.

I return to the pharmacy, insert my credit card in exchange for the original, now very expensive insulin, and return home with the promise of a refund once the pre-authorization goes through. I shoot off an email to my son's physician requesting her help. "Take your time," I write her. "We won't be home again for two weeks."

You know the drill. You've done it a hundred times, as have I. You have a plan for your day and the pharmacy is just stop number three on a six-stop day of errands. You've mapped it all out. Choreographed every step so as not to waste time or fuel, and certainly not to leave medicine in your 120-degrees Fahrenheit car on a blistering hot July day. Ten minutes in the pharmacy become fifteen, twenty, thirty minutes, and it's not their fault; but after half an hour you walk out with no medicine and a to-do list of phone calls to make and emails to send.

Situations like this are powerful enough to unhinge me. Like a tree bending under the weight of hurricane-force winds, unexpected obstacles to my caregiving can easily sway my mood. I don't like this behavior I see in myself. It tells me the disease has power not just over my son, but also over me.

I yearn to be stronger than my son's disease. I want to model true strength for him. In the T1D world, we often quote Bob Marley's famous line, "You never know how strong you are until being strong is your only choice." I know I don't have the luxury of being weak or relaxed in managing my son's condition, but what does true strength actually look like?

Why do I allow the interruptions to irritate me so much? If I'm honest, I judge a day that goes to plan as inherently superior to a day whose plans unravel. I define my own strength based on what I've accomplished or whether I had the wits to untangle all the surprises knotting up the timeline of my day. I think I mistake strength for being in control. But maybe being strong doesn't look like having it all together. Could true strength be found in a deep satisfaction that I'm loving well and doing the best I can?

My mother-in-law sent me a birthday card this year on which she wrote these words by Moses, the ancient Hebrew leader, "Satisfy me in the morning with your unfailing love that I may sing for joy and be glad all day."[3] I can't get the words out of my mind. What does it take for me to be satisfied? How can love keep me anchored in satisfaction and joy? What kind of deep inner satisfaction allows me to rejoice and be glad all day long, regardless of the interruptions that come my way?

I want to be strong enough that my inner satisfaction isn't contingent upon my day going just as I had planned. I don't want my son's illness to control me any more than I want it to control him.

---

3   Psalm 90:14.

What might it look like for me to change the way I define *strong*? What if instead of counting my accomplishments on a day that runs smoothly, I measured the *attitudes* I carry with me every day—including the days of interrupted plans? How might I begin to measure strength by the way I move through the storms of life with grace and courage rather than impatience and irritation?

To prevent unexpected challenges from controlling me begins by remembering that *how* I respond is a *choice* I make. Will I choose to offer understanding or annoyance? My bad attitudes won't resolve simply by wishing them away. It requires focused effort not to erupt when an unforeseen complication demands our attention. Personally, I pray regularly for wisdom to recognize when my irritation is building and self-control to resist engaging with anger. I take a few deep breaths in the moment to remind myself to stay calm. And I acknowledge that my example of kindness and self-control under pressure is itself a witness to hope.

There is much at stake here. I'm not the only one who needs to learn patience; I must teach my son to be patient with his healthcare needs. He has a long road ahead of him, years of managing the complexities of T1D as an adult. By showing him appropriate responses to dealing with the unforeseen interruptions of managing his healthcare, he will learn that impatience and anger are not the best responses.

I discover a deeper sense of peace as I embrace this new perspective. If I can release the self-imposed verdict of "failure" over a day that holds more interruptions than accomplishments checked off a to-do list, what remains? I see a parent who is determined to protect her child in every way she can. I see a mama-warrior who foregoes her own agenda so she can fight the battles that threaten her child.

When everything else is stripped away, I see love standing tall and strong.

Real strength lies not in managing to live a well-ordered life, avoiding all the swirling chaos, but in discovering beauty amidst the disorder.

I used to think being *strong* meant having all of life's uncertainties go according to my carefully orchestrated plans. I'm beginning to define *strong* differently. *Strong* means the ability to carry on even when things don't go to plan. *Strong* means the ability to move through life without grumbling or complaining when you have every reason to be discontent. *Strong* means not expecting life will turn out your way, and yet being able to reflect boldness and courage amidst the disappointing times.

Real strength lies not in managing to live a well-ordered life, avoiding all the swirling chaos, but in discovering beauty amidst the disorder.

Heart to Heart

- *How do you tend to handle the unforeseen situations of your caregiving life?*

- *In what ways does your child's disease make you feel weaker? Stronger?*

- *In what ways do you model strength to your child?*

PART THREE

The Two of Us

Chapter Ten

Stigma

The first condition of hope is to believe that you will have a future;
the second is to believe that there will be a decent world in which to live it.
—SCOTT RUSSELL SANDERS

"When will I get my bracelet?" Austin asks me, his bright eyes rimmed with long, feathery eyelashes locking mine.

"I ordered it last week. It should arrive any day now," I reply, relieved as I observe his enthusiasm for wearing a Medic Alert bracelet. I wasn't sure if he would balk at wearing a bracelet indicating he now has T1D.

There were eight children in his Montessori class in Connecticut, three of whom wore Medic Alert bracelets for their severe peanut allergies. Two of these children, Kyle and Julian, happened to be Austin's two best friends. For Austin, wearing the little silver bracelet with the red emblem in the shape of a snake wrapped around a staff was like putting on a fraternity pin. It indicated his kinship with his best friends.

These two boys set an example for my son of living courageously with a life-threatening condition. Every time either of these friends wanted to eat even the smallest piece of food he would run to his mother and ask for her permission. My son observed this behavior so frequently that it no longer seemed unusual to him. Now Austin must also seek my permission, and a shot of insulin, for every piece of food he eats. I'm thankful his two friends normalized this new routine for him.

The bracelet finally arrives, and I slip it on Austin's slender wrist. He misses his friends from Connecticut, but somehow this little bracelet is a link connecting them across the miles. He doesn't mind wearing it—he looked forward to it—because while it singles him out from among most of his peers, it identifies him as being like the two friends he left behind.

Many years have passed since Austin first wore the silver Medic Alert bracelet with the red painted emblem. He now wears a more discreet rubber bracelet indicating that he lives with T1D.

I open my email from diaTribe, one of my favorite online diabetes resources. The title of the lead article intrigues me: "The Numbers of Shame and Blame: How Stigma Affects Patients and Diabetes Management." Over the years Austin's attitudes regarding T1D have shifted. It's not simply his choice of a medical bracelet that has changed. Increasingly, he pays less and less attention to his disease despite his growing responsibility for managing it. My desire to keep him healthy and safe is now in constant tension with his desire to live without thinking about diabetes.

I should have known his sense of ease over being different from his peers wouldn't last forever. For almost seven years he remained mostly nonchalant about the disease. He rarely complained about the challenges he faced and didn't show signs of embarrassment or shame because of it. But with the increase in self-awareness so typical of pre-adolescence, Austin eventually grew tired of being different from his friends. He became irritable if I had to help him with his infusion site changes. Almost overnight, the bracelet became an annoying encumbrance. All he wanted was to be "normal."

I begin reading the article. "A 2014 study by the diaTribe Foundation found that diabetes stigma affects 76% of people living with T1D and 83% of parents raising a child with T1D."[4]

I can't believe what I'm reading. The statistics are *so high*.

Stigma. The word itself sounds uncomfortable on my lips. Quickly I look up the dictionary definition of stigma, just to be sure I understand what I'm reading. A stigma is defined as "a sense of disgrace associated with a particular circumstance, quality, or person. It's also defined as a set of negative and often unfair beliefs that a society or group of people have about something." So in my son's case, diabetes stigma is both the sense of shame he may feel, as well as the set of negative beliefs others have about him and the disease.

The article continues. "The majority of respondents who believe T1D is associated with social stigma identified the top three drivers of diabetes stigma—a perception of failure of personal responsibility, a perception of being a burden on society, and a perception of having a character flaw."[5]

I cringe as I read these findings. Not many diseases carry the same weight of shame and blame as T1D. I know that. I've been surrounded by the disease my entire life, so I've witnessed the shame and blame firsthand. But still, the findings haunt me.

Does my son feel like he's a failure when his blood sugars don't cooperate and do what he wants them to do? Maybe he does. I know as his parent and caregiver I feel like a failure when his A1C—the measure of his three-month average blood sugar—isn't what I had hoped it would be. Does he feel like he's a burden on society? On his school? On his family? Oh, I hope not. I can hardly even reread that last driver of stigma

---

4 "The Numbers of Shame and Blame: How Stigma Affects Patients and Diabetes Management," diatribe.org, Aug. 7, 2014, https://diatribe.org/issues/67/learning-curve.

5 Ibid.

on the list. Does he feel like he has a *character flaw* simply because he has T1D? My heart rises up to my throat.

When we live in a world so obsessed with picture-perfect health, beauty, and body image, it's easy to see yourself as damaged goods when you live with chronic illness.

How can I help my son navigate living with chronic illness in such a way that he doesn't fall prey to the shame and failure associated with disease stigma? Rereading the statistics, I pause and ask myself another question. How do I as his parent carry disease stigma? The survey tells me 83 percent of us parents raising a child with T1D are affected by it. Am I a part of that 83 percent? When his physician suggests we make some changes to achieve better outcomes, do my reactions model for my son my own feelings of failure, guilt, or shame?

Whether we talk about it or not, stigma deeply affects most people living with T1D and many other chronic diseases. Diabetes stigma drives feelings of failure, guilt, shame, blame, embarrassment, and isolation. Trying to manage a disease that has so many variables affecting it is like trying to pick up fallen autumn leaves in a windstorm.

With a complex disease to manage, both the caregiver and the child have to focus on many objectives simultaneously. If we're not careful with our language, we can pepper our children with a steady stream of target goals all beginning with the word *should*. Feelings of failure, guilt, shame, blame, embarrassment, and isolation are the offspring of a lifetime of unfulfilled *shoulds*.

Feelings of failure, guilt, shame, blame, embarrassment, and isolation are the offspring of a lifetime of unfulfilled shoulds.

Like the seasoned orchestra conductor interrupting a rehearsal when he detects one false note among the ninety performers, I can often focus all my attention on the one problem I want my son to address among all the things he's doing right. I don't even mention what he's doing well; I just zero in like a laser beam on the one thing that needs improvement. I've heard that for every negative comment we give someone, we need to make at least five positive comments to counterbalance the effect of the criticism. Why, when I know this to be true, do I continue to harp on what my son could do better, rather than focus my energy on praising what he has done well?

It's hard work paying such close attention to my attitudes and language. But I realize more is at stake here than my "getting everything right" as I oversee his care. Yes, I want to teach him how to manage his disease, but it's much more important that I offer him words of love and support every day. I hold my son's tender life in my hands, and the messages I convey—both spoken and unspoken—about who he is despite the disease really do matter.

I don't want my words to contribute to his feelings of failure or shame. Instead, I want to help him recognize the voice of shame as a lie and teach him to refuse to give into its power. We help our children break free from shame when we model for them that we are no longer held in its grip.

I'm learning to pay attention to how I carry stigma so as not to project my own feelings of failure and shame onto my son. When he was little, I was in charge of every decision related to his care. If the endocrinologist was pleased with my son's blood sugar readings during the prior three months, I was proud—of both my son and me. When the results were not as the doctor or I had hoped, I felt like a failure. Like a bad mother. I felt judged. But maybe I was just judging myself. I told myself I had to try harder because my son's health and life were at stake. Sometimes the prospect of improved outcomes felt hopeless despite my best efforts.

I understand the feelings of diabetes stigma. The 83 percent is me.

As hard as it is for me, that means not treating the results of my son's medical appointments like my report card. When I express feelings of failure and shame if the doctor encourages us to work harder at managing my son's care, I teach my child to be ashamed if he doesn't hit his targets. My message becomes *your value is in your results*, as if the way he manages his disease has some moral implication on his life.

That's not the message I want my child to receive from me. I want my message to be this: *You are wonderfully and perfectly made, just the way you are, and nothing will ever change my love for you.* For my child to hear that message instead of the voice of shame, I need to be committed to a habit of open communication with him.

Our children may be surprised when they first experience feelings of disease stigma. We can help them by creating safe spaces for them to express their feelings. Generally that means being willing to open up with them first, sharing our feelings with them. When I tell my child how the disease makes me feel, I give him permission to share his own feelings. Open-ended "what" and "how" questions tend to be most effective at engaging even quiet children to go beyond a yes-no answer.

I'm realizing my responsibility doesn't end with managing the effect of disease stigma on just my son or me. I'm also invited to play a part in changing the larger community's perception of a person living with chronic illness. All too often, people not experienced with my son's condition begin conversations with this disclaimer, "You know more about this than I do," and they continue by offering all kinds of unsolicited advice. Inevitably, despite my efforts at explaining the complexity of the disease, I will be told that because my son *looks* so good and takes his insulin, he will be *just fine*. I imagine you've experienced these conversations as well and find it just as frustrating to be on the receiving end of unsolicited, inaccurate advice.

Stigma apparently includes society's inaccurate belief that chronic illness is not so bad as long as you still look good on the outside.

As my mother used to say, "Pick your battles." Sometimes, no matter how I respond, the person I'm speaking to will not accept the reality of my child's disease. It's better to change the topic than risk increased frustration with this type of person. But when I engage with people who actually choose to listen and learn, I can use my voice to educate them about the complexity of my child's disease. With them I can share how hard my son works to stay healthy and strong, all the while being clear we're not looking for pity. On a larger scale, I can use my pen to dispel myths about the disease and spread truth instead. I can get involved with local or online organizations in the T1D space, thereby magnifying my efforts for a broader reach.

My hope for a better world for my son, one in which he doesn't feel stigmatized, begins with me. When I change my own views about the disease, I experience the freedom of living outside the labels of failure, shame, and blame, and can offer that same freedom to my son. And if we can change our viewpoint, I hold out hope that the larger community can as well.

Heart to Heart

- *How have you or your child experienced disease stigma?*

- *What changes in perspective, language, and behavior could you make to help your child feel less stigmatized?*

- *How might you help the larger community be more accepting of your child's condition?*

Chapter Eleven

Fatigue

"Hope" is the thing with feathers
That perches in the soul
And sings the tune without the words
And never stops—at all.
—Emily Dickinson

When my son was little, I had one goal in mind for his overall well-being—to let him live as much like other kids as possible. That one goal informed many of the decisions I made regarding his care. I couldn't take the disease away from him, but at least I could carry some of the burden for him.

Every day brought a host of disease-related decisions and activities with it. There were decisions regarding food choices and their carbohydrate and fat values. There were decisions about how much insulin to deliver based on what he ate, how much he had exercised or was going to exercise, if he was fighting a virus, or if he was traveling and sitting still for a long time. Growth spurts meant a complete recalculation of all his insulin ratios, determined largely by trial and error. I interrupted him at least six times a day to check his blood sugar by finger stick, and every two to three days to change his insulin infusion site.

In the early years, I had to manage all my son's care because he was too young to safely manage things on his own. As he grew, he assumed progressively more responsibility for his care, but I still tried to carry as much of his diabetes burden as I could so he could live as carefree as possible. He would have his entire adult life to manage his diabetes, I reasoned.

Not all parents have this same goal in mind as their number one priority. For some, the goal is for their child to become independent as quickly as possible. This may be dictated by constraints within the family or by the clear desire of the child. There's no right or wrong approach. Every person is different, and every parent-child relationship is different. In my case, my son was happy to let me handle as much of the decision-making as I could so he could get on with being a kid. Perhaps your child doesn't have a disease like T1D and will never be able to live independently. I know disease fatigue is especially real for you, as it was for me for many years.

Whether or not your child's care requires the magnitude and complexity of decision-making as T1D, every disease carries with it a large share of decisions. There's research to read, treatment options to weigh, doctors to interview, hospitals to evaluate, observations to make regarding fine-tuning treatment protocols, troubleshooting, and of course the challenge of living with the decisions we make.

A few years after my son was diagnosed, I read a statement by an endocrinologist that deeply impacted me. *More than any other disease, the primary caregiver of a child with T1D is responsible for multiple life-saving decisions on a daily basis.* My new responsibility terrified me. Making all those decisions might be tolerable if the disease would cooperate with us. However, T1D is notoriously unpredictable, as outcomes often don't follow predictable patterns based on inputs. Best intentions don't guarantee good results when trying to manage certain diseases.

Some days I grew so weary of being the caregiver. Life itself felt like a battle, and I was worn out from the fight. And I wasn't even the one living with the disease. Often I wanted to cry and scream and pound my fists at the inconsistency of it all. T1D is an unrelenting, uncooperative disease that rarely responds as directed.

When the disease was most unpredictable, the stress and fatigue would lead me to tears. These were private moments, not shared with anyone other than my husband. I had made a decision to be a strong support for my son. If I needed to be his cheerleader, then cheer I would. If I needed to be his chief mathematician—counting carbohydrates and dosing insulin—then math would be my new favorite subject.

When our children are small and we carry much of the disease burden for them, we naturally experience disease fatigue as well. For many of us, the day will come when our fatigue ends, as the management of the disease becomes fully our child's responsibility. That's when we must be prepared to help if their fatigue becomes burnout.

We finish loading the final boxes and bags from his college dorm room into my Toyota SUV and gently place his Taylor guitar on top of it all. How could one young man and his roommate squeeze so much stuff into that tiny room? Summer vacation has officially begun, and I can't wait to have my son home with me for three whole months.

When my children were young, bedtime was always the best time for heart-to-heart conversations. Somehow, in the dark of night, in the safety of sheets and blankets and duvets, the deep concerns of the day would come spilling out. Now that my son is older, our conversations in the dark have been replaced by conversations in the car. Perhaps it's the guarantee that no one will interrupt us or eavesdrop on what he has to say. Perhaps the safety of the car reminds him of the safety of his childhood bedroom. Or maybe he has just bottled up his emotions long enough and can't wait until we get home to share them with me.

Pleasant and cheerful as we pack up his belongings, he gives me no indication anything is troubling him. We barely make it to the highway before he releases the burdens pent up in his heart.

"I'm so tired of never feeling well," he begins. "I'm always sick. I don't know anyone else who has endured as much illness as I have."

As he is not one prone to self-pity, this is new language for my son. I know his words are true, and I want to affirm what he feels. I also want to discover if there's something else going on.

"I'm so sorry, honey. I know it's difficult," I offer. "Did something happen to make you feel this way?"

Tears well up in his eyes as he shares with me his private fatigue of fighting for his health for such a long time. He pauses before continuing.

"I haven't felt well since I was five years old."

His words stab me in the heart. I've never heard him speak like this before. Obviously, I know his life is harder than any of his friends' lives, but he has never led me so deeply into his private pain before now. He always let on that diabetes was no big deal. As his tears begin to flow alongside his words, I see for the first time the weight of everything he has carried for fifteen long years.

I know there have been times since his diagnosis when he has felt "well," at least for a few moments or hours. But I don't contradict him. I hear and receive what he tells me—not a day has gone by that his body hasn't felt the effects of living with T1D. Every time he eats, he feels the effect of rising blood sugar. Every time he exercises, he feels the effect of falling blood sugar. Whenever he's sick or stressed or growing, he feels the effect of swinging blood sugar. Indeed, every day he feels the physical toll of this disease on his body. And every day he also must deal with the psychological burden of making myriad decisions regarding his health to try to manage a very unmanageable disease.

In many ways I understand his burnout. It has only been a few years since I managed his care and regularly experienced caregiver fatigue. I may not have felt the physical effects of the disease in my body, but I felt keenly the emotional fatigue from carrying the weight of the complex decisions I had to make. I had hoped my efforts at shouldering much of my young child's burden would have protected him from burnout and fatigue as he grew.

I'm concerned to see my son so defeated. Burnout often leads to feelings of hopelessness that result in dangerously compromised levels of self-care.

How can I help my son hold onto hope in these seasons of fatigue? Do my words of encouragement make any difference? When he's more in need of a cure—or at least a vacation from T1D—than a pep talk, does a hug or a kind word really make any difference?

I choose to believe they do make a difference. I choose to believe in the power of hope expressed through love. In desperate times like these, I must hold ever tighter to hope so I can guide my child back to its secure embrace. I can no longer carry the disease for him, but I can lift his head and point him toward hope.

I must hold ever tighter to hope so I can
guide my child back to its secure embrace.
I can no longer carry the disease for him,
but I can lift his head and point him toward hope.

Hope requires the belief that as bad as things may be, they will not always remain the same. If, as Emily Dickinson wrote, *hope is the thing with feathers,* then hope is meant to lift us up. Like a bird taking flight, hope has the power to transport us to a vision of a better tomorrow.

Where burnout declares *you alone carry this burden,* I sow seeds of hope by communicating to my son that I am still in his corner as his greatest champion. Hope says to my son, "Keep going, keep fighting, keep believing, and don't give up." While I'm no longer his caregiver, I'm still here as his coach, mentor, and cheerleader. He is not alone.

I create space for hope to flourish when I'm careful enough with my words that I don't contribute to his feelings of disease stigma or failure. There's a delicate balance to maintain here. My adult son can easily perceive my attempts at giving him one more piece of advice regarding his care as overbearing. When my words appear judgmental, I stamp out hope before it has a chance to take root.

Into the hopelessness that asserts *my life will always be this difficult,* hope glimmers when I invite my child to talk about his frustration with the disease. Often he prefers to stay silent, but if he chooses to share his thoughts with me, I can receive what he says without judging or trying to fix things. I pray with him, releasing the burden to his God and mine. And we seek professional help when the challenges are greater than we can handle together.

I ride on the wings of hope when I see advances to my son's care. Treatments for his disease have improved significantly since he was first diagnosed. Of course I wish there were a cure today, but when I see progress accelerating, I believe his life will be even better in the years to come.

Hope is not the guarantee that things will get easier,
just the prospect that they might.

I choose to live in hope for my child's future. Hope is not the guarantee that things will get easier, just the prospect that they might. Hope tells me to keep looking up and reminds me to live in love. When I live in love, I invite my son into a life of hope.

Heart to Heart

- *How have you experienced fatigue from managing your child's care?*

- *How have you responded to signs of your child's disease fatigue?*

- *How might you invite hope into your places of fatigue and burnout? Into your child's fatigue and burnout?*

Chapter Twelve

Encourage

"Come, Mr. Frodo!" he cried. "I can't carry it for you,
but I can carry you and it as well."
—J.R.R. Tolkien

I'm not known as one who frequently leaves her family to go on a "girls' weekend." Which is to say, I had never left my family for a girls' weekend before. But when the invitation came to get away to the beach for an early fall weekend with my dearest friends from college, my heart leapt at the chance to finally say yes to a little personal time away.

These were my best friends from college. We had chosen to live with, or next to, one another all four years during our college experience. We lived through all of each other's highs and lows during those years yet sailed off after graduation into our own adult lives, only keeping up with one another by occasional calls, visits, texts, and our college reunions. Gathered around the table at our thirtieth reunion, we vowed to remedy our past pattern and see one another more frequently. Most of us had children in college—there were only a couple of children still in the nest—so it was the perfect time to have an extended visit together.

It feels so odd to experience this sense of freedom. For thirteen years I have been my son's primary caregiver for all things related to diabetes.

For thirteen years I never would have dreamed of leaving him overnight unless I had put in place every imaginable safety net.

But he's a college freshman now. I'm no longer there to catch him when his blood sugars fall. My schedule is no longer intricately interwoven with his. And so I gladly accepted the invitation to spend a few days at the beach.

The call comes on Sunday morning, about 10 a.m. Mothers should delight in seeing their phone light up with their child's number, but I know my son well enough to understand that a Sunday morning call from him would be no how-ya-doin' call. It would be a call for help. And my heart skips a beat.

"Hi darling, how are you?" I say, steeling myself for what is to come.

"I've run out of insulin." That's all he needs to say for me to know he's in real trouble. "I ordered it, but I forgot to pick it up from the pharmacy this week."

In a world with diabetes, insulin is my son's lifeline; how could he have no more insulin? He tells me how much is left in his insulin pump, and I quickly calculate. There's not enough insulin for breakfast. If he doesn't eat anything, he has only a couple hours of insulin left.

And that's going to be a big problem. The pharmacy he uses at college is a small family-owned business and is closed on Sundays. His insulin can't be purchased without a prescription, and my son's prescription is literally locked up and will be inaccessible for the next twenty-two hours. When the pharmacy reopens the following morning, it will be about nineteen hours too late.

The next hour is a blur of phone calls to CHOP—the Children's Hospital of Philadelphia—waiting for the on-call fellow to return my call, getting special approval from the insurance company to process another order of insulin—since his order had already been filled but not picked up—finding another pharmacy, and finding transportation for Austin to get to the pharmacy. Back and forth the calls and texts fly until it is settled and I can breathe again.

It was an innocent mistake, but innocent mistakes can prove costly when you have a life-threatening disease. It takes all my strength not to holler and hurl my insulting judgments at him. How could he be so careless? I smolder with indignation. Haven't I warned him a million times to keep an eye on his supplies? Doesn't he understand he put himself in an extremely dangerous situation today?

Why won't he just do what I ask him to do? He must know what I have taught him and what I ask of him is for his own good. He must know it is all to protect him.

I long to take the easy road, to let go of restraint and release a steady stream of reminders of what could happen if he does...what could happen if he doesn't... I want to yell and scream and push my mama weight around. I don't want to guard my temper. I want to release it. Release it all on him until he understands how serious this is, for today and for his future.

I stand, shaking in my anger. And in that moment, like scales falling from my eyes, I see the overwhelming fear I carry, each and every day of my son's life. I am not walking in freedom but living in bondage to all the potential landmines of this disease. I see the risks and declare a judgment of *fragile* over my son's life. I live locked in the assurance that because of disease, my son's life is more fragile than the lives of his siblings.

But is it really? Why do I think disease is the only arbiter of life and death? Do I have authority to proclaim life and death over my children? Am I God? Do I know the number of hairs on my children's heads? Do I know the number of days appointed to any one of them?

I have made bedfellows with fear, but I do not slip under the covers naked. I have clothed myself once again with my need for control, as if by controlling every unforeseen problem I can ensure a smooth road ahead. I insist on attempting to control the myriad decisions that have far-reaching consequences affecting my son's health. How I long to slay the two giants of fear and control, but I seem to keep spiraling back to them.

How I long to slay the two giants of fear and control,
but I seem to keep spiraling back to them.

I tell myself that I teach my son because I want him to know all I have learned about managing this disease. Let me speak truth. I teach my son because I want him to manage this disease *exactly* as I would, and in so doing, help me keep up the illusion that I am in control of life and death.

But I am not God. And I am not in control of life and death.

I never thought it would be this difficult. I had accepted that having children meant I could not control their thoughts or decisions any more than I could control their height or hair color. Pregnant with my first child, I pondered at length the maxim "to have a child is to decide forever to have your heart go walking around outside your body." I let its full weight wash over me, knowing my heart would break many times over the physical and emotional pain my children would experience in life.

Parenting always involves a walk of faith; the journey is just a little harder if your child shares life with a chronic illness.

There are days, like today, when I tire of playing the role of encourager. I don't want to think creatively and spin this into a positive and encouraging learning experience. I just want to get my own way and control the outcomes of my son's choices. Because the frontal lobe of the human brain doesn't fully attach until around age twenty-five, my teenage son isn't influenced by the fear of future consequences arising from poor decisions he makes today. Until then, his focus is centered on things around him—his friends, family, academics, faith, sports, and other activities. Without the fully adult capacity for future thinking, he can't be expected to be as motivated as I am to maintain good health.

My mind drifts back to the face of my son. I remember he is only eighteen years old. He doesn't live in the place of constant fear for his future. He lives in the place of endless possibility. And that is exactly what I want for him. I really don't want his every thought to be about this disease. I really don't want him to obsess over fears about his future. I want him to live and dream and thrive and soar.

Ultimately, my son is his own person who will make his own decisions. When I choose to yell at him for his carelessness or for making decisions that differ from what I would choose, I shut down our communication and may lose the privilege of supporting him. When I choose to live in the bondage of fear for my son's future, I am choosing death over life. When I choose anger and bitterness over kindness and forgiveness, I am choosing death over life. When I choose selfishness and control over love, I am choosing death over life.

I pull out my phone to send him one more text.

"Are you okay now, honey?"

"Yeah, I put in a new cartridge of insulin."

"Did you get anything to eat?"

"I will, once the insulin brings my blood sugar back down."

"Okay, good. I'm glad it all worked out."

My role is to teach, to influence, to encourage. To encourage literally means to *fill* him with *courage*. Courage to make the best decisions for his body. Courage that will protect him from constant fear about his future. The responsibility is mine to encourage him to live his best life today, while teaching him how to care for his body as well as he can. Mine is to model for him a life of trust and not a life of fear. Mine is to teach, looking for opportunities among the failures and setbacks and triumphs to lovingly show him just a little bit more. Mine is always to give him a second, a third, a fourth chance, lavishing on him grace upon grace.

My phone lights up one more time. I press on the text from my son. "Thanks Mom."

"You're welcome. I love you."

"Love you too."

Heart to Heart

- *What is your go-to response when your child doesn't make wise choices for himself? Is it anger and yelling? Storming away? Pity? Sympathy? Encouragement?*

- *In what ways might your responses when under stress negatively or positively influence your child's outlook for her future?*

- *How might you modify your language with your child so you can fill him with courage and hope, even in a crisis?*

Chapter Thirteen

Trust

The best way to find out if you can trust somebody is to trust them.
—ERNEST HEMINGWAY

I've never been much of a baker. Cooking nice dinners is more to my liking. Baking involves all the precision of a chemistry experiment, whereas cooking allows for the improv of a jazz trio. Besides, once T1D came into our lives it didn't feel right to spend time baking sweet treats that were sure to elevate my son's blood sugar.

But Christmastime was the one exception to this pattern. Every Christmas I would stock up on little yellow packages of Toll House morsels, fresh five-pound bags of sugar and flour, raisins, old-fashioned oats, and butter. Lots of butter. Some years I managed to make a few varieties of Christmas cookies; other years the holiday season would come and go with one lone item remaining on my Christmas to-do list: Make Christmas Cookies.

This was one of those years. The season moved too fast, or I moved too slowly, and the bag of chocolate chips remained unopened, abandoned on the pantry shelf. My eye occasionally caught sight of the bright yellow bag when I went to the pantry to fetch a box of crackers or a jar of pasta sauce. Sometimes I would scold myself just a little bit for not finding the time to bake those Christmas cookies for my kids.

We're having pasta for dinner tonight. I head toward the pantry, where, reaching for a box of penne, I can't help noticing the bag of chocolate chips. It has been opened, the ripped end now sloppily folded back to give the appearance of being closed.

I pause a moment to remember if I opened the bag sometime in the prior few months. No. I would have placed the entire opened bag in a large Ziploc bag to keep the chips fresh and keep any hungry pests out. *Who got into the chocolate chips? It must have been Alexander or Alicia who opened the bag,* I conclude. *Austin doesn't sneak food. I'll have to speak with them about not leaving open bags of food in the pantry—it's an invitation for pantry pests and leaves me without enough chips to make a full cookie recipe.*

First, I ask Alexander, then Alicia. Both children assure me they didn't touch the chocolate chips. We have always practiced honesty in our home, so I take them at their word.

"It couldn't be Austin," I tell myself in disbelief. "He always shows me what he eats so I can count the carbohydrates." I know that children with T1D reach a point when they no longer need their parent to estimate carbohydrate values and dose insulin for them as they begin to do more for themselves. But we're not at that stage yet. Austin is only eight years old. My heart begins to race as I process the likelihood that Austin is secretly eating food without telling me. It can become dangerous pretty quickly if I make insulin-dosing decisions based on inaccurate information regarding his food consumption.

Austin flies through the back door, sweaty and breathless from shooting hoops in the driveway, his full head of long blond hair glued to his wet forehead. "Austin," I begin, before he can run off again. "I noticed the bag of chocolate chips was opened in the pantry. Did you get into them without asking me?"

"Oh, yeah," he answers nonchalantly. "I wanted some chocolate."

I don't know which surprises me more—that he was immediately honest with me, or that he suddenly thought he could eat chocolate without needing to take insulin! "Austin," I continue, "you remember that I need to know *everything* you eat so I can be sure to give you the correct amount of insulin, right?"

He nods his head. "Uh-huh."

"Have you been sneaking food a lot?" I venture cautiously.

"No. I just wanted some chocolate the other day," he replies casually.

I breathe a sigh of relief before continuing. "If you want some chocolate, just tell me and I can work it in and give you insulin for it. If I don't know you've eaten something, I won't know why your blood sugar is high later, and that could lead me to make changes to your insulin regimen that could hurt you. Do you understand?"

He nods his head again. "Yeah. Sorry."

In a flash, my blond boy is back outside, and all I can hear through the closed door is the sound of the basketball bouncing on the driveway.

Building relationships within my family based on the three-legged stool of trust, honesty, and respect has always been important to me. Remove any one of these qualities and love struggles to be our family's guiding force. I had no way of knowing as a young parent how crucial these tenets of a healthy family would be for us once chronic illness became a part of our life. The stakes are so much higher now. Reduce honesty, and I no longer have all the facts to make informed decisions regarding my son's care. Take away respect, and communication between my child and me breaks down. Trust is essential for effective collaboration to take place.

Trust between us begins with demonstrating to my child that I am trustworthy. My child learns to be honest with me according to the model of honesty I live out for him. Over time my son has learned I don't lie to him. He has also observed I don't round the edges of truth with other people either, even when it's tempting, and sometimes easier, to tell a slightly revised version of the truth. When our children hear us lie—even just a little white lie—they learn to tell us whatever version of the truth is the least likely to get them into trouble. Trust within a family stands on the shoulders of honesty.

Trust within a family stands on the shoulders of honesty.

Dishonesty isn't the only enemy of a healthy family. Sarcasm hurts familial relationships because it tears down respect. When we're frustrated with our child's level of self-care, a common tactic is to lace our words with sarcasm in an attempt to hide what we really feel. But underneath every sarcastic remark is an element of criticizing truth. Words are important. They're a reflection of the heart. And yet often in the comfort of our own family life, and under the pressure of chronic disease, we forget to be careful with our words.

Some days, when the disease doesn't respond as I expect it will, the temptation is great to take out my frustration on my son. I struggle against the urge to interrogate him, scold him, or scream at the very disease itself. How does that help my son?

Sometimes I forget how vulnerable he must feel. He has to rely on me for so much more than his siblings do. He must get annoyed having me survey and approve everything he eats, coming to me for insulin every time he's hungry, and asking for glucose whenever his blood sugar drops too low. He doesn't like this arrangement any more than I do. I want him to know I'll always be there to carry *his* frustration without insisting he carry mine.

As I demonstrate that I'm trustworthy, respectful, and honest with him and others, my son learns he can trust me implicitly. This helps him develop his own patterns of honest and respectful behavior. As our children take on more of their own self-care, open communication between them and us is essential. As they grow, the issues will no longer simply be about open bags of chocolate chips—as important as accurate carb counting may be. Our conflicts will revolve around more complex decisions regarding diet, exercise, parties, and alcohol. And we'll need honesty and trust between us to navigate these conversations with love and respect. Open communication doesn't happen overnight; it develops slowly, over time, with conversations marinated in trust and mutual respect.

Perhaps trust and honesty have already broken down in your relationship with your child and the idea of developing mutual respect between you seems hopeless. When my relationship with my son feels damaged in some way, I usually begin by apologizing to him, acknowledging my part in the problem, and asking him for a fresh start. I also evaluate the deeper issues in my heart—like fear, control, and fatigue—and seek to understand how they might be influencing my behavior. Asking my son for a do-over allows us to begin building trust anew.

Fostering honest, trusting relationships with our children doesn't guarantee they will always be honest with us, especially during their teenage years. But cultivating honesty and openness with our children before they reach adolescence, by repeatedly laying down roots of trust, gives us the best chance at enjoying a healthy relationship with them as they grow.

As I create an environment for my son to trust me, we also create avenues for me to trust him. As he grows and more of the T1D management falls on his shoulders, I have to trust him enough to *get out of the way*, allowing him to manage things on his own. Trusting my son to do his part protects me from my tendency to hover too much and nag him to do things my way. Trust, it seems, is a two-way street.

Heart to Heart

• *How do you intentionally foster trust, honesty, and respect in your relationship with your child?*

• *What changes might you consider making in your language or attitudes to encourage mutual trust to grow between you?*

• *If trust is breaking down in your relationship, what steps could you take to rebuild it?*

Chapter Fourteen

Let's Make a Deal

Give, but give until it hurts.
—MOTHER TERESA

It was time to change my son's insulin therapy routine. I asked our medical team about insulin pump therapy, but their response was always the same. "Your son must be on shots for at least two years before we'll consider him for insulin pump therapy." Knowing an insulin pump would give my ever hungry seven-year-old son greater flexibility in eating, I asked every three months for approval. Yet visit after visit they told me to wait. And so, like a teenager shopping for a prom gown one year too early, I researched all the pumps and what they offered. With great enthusiasm I shared everything I discovered with my son.

I was so excited. He was horrified.

"You'll be able to eat all your meals and snacks without getting a shot," I explained. "The pump will deliver your insulin through the attached tubing. All we have to do is input a carbohydrate value into the pump."

My son made no response and barely looked me in the eye.

I pressed on. "It will be like getting one big shot every two to three days when we change the insulin pump site, instead of four to seven small shots a day. Won't that be so nice?"

He didn't think it sounded very nice at all.

To be clear, my son certainly didn't like getting four to seven shots of insulin a day, but he had gotten used to it and accepted that this was how things would be. The thought of changing his routine from shots to a pump was terrifying to him *because it was new*.

I should have known he wouldn't be enthusiastic about making a change to his routine. I had tried the year before switching him from insulin syringes to the much more discreet insulin pens, and he had balked at the idea of changing his established routine.

Accepting change can be difficult. It's hard to modify a course of treatment—even if we're not particularly fond of the current treatment. We come to trust the protocol, looking to it to keep us safe. My son seems to take everything in stride, accepting the rigors of living with this disease without much complaint, so it's easy for me to forget he's using all his mental energy just to accept the way things are.

We know the one living with chronic illness needs courage to face the challenges of their disease, but parents also need courage. We need courage to embrace our role as the wiser parent figure. It's our responsibility to anticipate the bumps that will come in the road—especially when we're asking our child to accept *change*—and to navigate those bumps with courage, grace, and confidence.

Any time we ask our child to change a routine they have finally accepted is a time for potential eruption. Some days I don't want to enter into the fight to convince my child the new way really is the better way. Some days it's easier to accept the status quo and leave things as they are, even if I believe it's not the best way. Some days I just don't want to enter into the long battle of convincing my child that mama really does know best.

As much as we might want to take the path of least resistance, it's important not to walk away from our responsibility to influence our child's thoughts and behaviors for the better. They might not readily admit it, but our children look to us for guidance—not as some authoritarian figure demanding his or her own way, but as a wise parent with enough life experience to light the way for them.

The greatest gift we can offer our children when a change in their medical care is required is to exercise our parental responsibility with love and understanding.

The greatest gift we can offer our children when a change in their medical care is required is to exercise our parental responsibility with love and understanding.

I was so excited for my son to have a better tool to manage this disease that I almost missed his cues. What I regarded as better tools he saw as frightening and potentially dangerous.

The day finally arrives. I have selected the insulin pump I think is best for my son, and we await the arrival of "the pump lady." She's coming to the house on that hot June day to start Austin on his new insulin pump.

We make our way over to the family room sofa, Austin sandwiched between the two grownups who are about to turn a seven-year-old's world upside down. His fidgeting begins, and I'm sure he's not focusing on what the pump lady is saying. *No matter*, I tell myself. *I'll be managing his pump for the first year or so anyway.*

She is kind and gentle with us. It's all so new and there's a lot to absorb. Austin continues to squirm—my energetic son has had to sit still for longer than he would like. She programs the pump with the settings we think are appropriate. She loads the pump with saline, which we will use for the first three days to practice. Next she fills the tubing just until we see tiny droplets of the liquid bead along the tip of the insertion device.

Looking up, she asks my son, "Where do you want to wear it? Your thigh, your arm, or your butt?"

Eyes wild and darting back and forth between the faces of the two grownups, his question pierces me with both its innocence and revelation of his loss of trust in me. "You want me to wear that thing?"

I thought I had explained everything so carefully. I thought I had reviewed every aspect of this new treatment to him and that he understood it. Clearly that was not the case. Clearly something was lost in translation, for he was in no way mentally prepared to have a six mm piece of plastic inserted into his flesh, through which the insulin would flow from twenty-four inches of tubing, that connected to his insulin pump, which he would now have to carry in a pouch around his waist 24/7.

It sounds complicated because it is complicated.

The tears pooling in his eyes like giant saucers tell me he wants nothing to do with my plans for improving his healthcare.

In an instant he is off the sofa, running up to his room, far from the two grownups and their crazy plans to make *his* life better.

Almost instinctively, I know this is not to become a battle of wills. It's so tempting to go nose to nose with people when we sense we're losing control of a situation. And it's all the more tempting to do when the one we're staring down is our child. Yet something tells me I am not to throw my mama weight around and force my seven-year-old to do as I say just because I'm bigger and older than he is. Like the flick of a light switch that illuminates a formerly dark room, I understand his fear of change.

I understand it because, for the first time, I choose to *feel* it rather than *dismiss* it.

My heart melts with love and compassion for my dear child. He did nothing to bring this disease on himself, and yet he has valiantly dealt with much added responsibility and restriction in these past two years. This change to his daily routine was my idea, not his, and it falls on me to conceive a way to help him see its possibilities.

The pump lady looks at me hard, her eyes saying what her lips will not. *How long will this mother let him stay up there? I have other people to see, after all, and can't stay here all afternoon.* My mind races to conceive a plan.

"Let me wear the pump," I tell her. "Insert the pump catheter into my flesh. I'll wear it and deliver the saline into my body every time I eat during these next three days. We can practice using the pump on me."

The pump lady agrees to my plan, and within minutes I feel the sting as the needle pierces my flesh. I have three days to convince Austin to try this new device.

Over the next three days, with perhaps too much enthusiasm, I show my son how easy the pump is to use. Every time I draw up a syringe of insulin to insert into the fleshy part of his arm, I point out that all I have to do is push a few buttons and the saline flows into my body without my even noticing it.

He's not impressed. Maybe I should have shown less excitement over a medical device.

With just hours to go in my little experiment, and no real sign that my son is interested in wearing the insulin pump, I pull him close to me and have one of the many mother-son, heart-to-heart conversations we would have over the years. I begin with honesty. With love. With a simple statement he is sure to understand.

"Honey, it's my responsibility as your parent to take care of you. Loving you and caring for you is one of the greatest joys of my life. But along with the joy of being your mama comes the responsibility of always trying to do what's best for you."

Does he know in that moment I'm talking about the insulin pump? If he does, he doesn't let on, nor does he shut me out.

"Do you know I always try to do what's best for you and I would never hurt you?" His big green eyes lock with mine, and he nods his head. Yes. Yes, he knows my love is real, so I press on with just a bit more courage.

"From what I have read and what I have learned, your blood sugars will be in much better control if you use a pump rather than shots. That's why I want you to try the pump. It's to keep you healthier, to keep you safe. As your mama, I always have to look for ways to keep you healthy and safe."

"Let's make a deal," I say to him. "Let's make a deal that if after six months there's no improvement in your average blood sugars, and you still don't like the pump, you don't have to keep using it. But if after six months your blood sugars are in better control on the pump, then we have to keep using it."

I exhale and look at his beautiful face, framed by the halo of blond silk. I have made my wager. Will he accept it? The silent moments tick into eternity.

"Okay."

That's it. That's all I get from my gentle son whose restored trust in his mama nearly breaks my heart.

Just one word. "Okay."

There was never another word spoken about the wisdom of using the insulin pump or the challenge of changing up his routine. We navigated those early days on the insulin pump together, as a team—I as the coach, he as the star player. He quickly came to enjoy the freedoms that the pump afforded him and never once asked to return to shots. Not even after those first six months when I asked him if he was content to continue using the pump.

And oh, by the way, his average blood sugars improved dramatically.

Heart to Heart

- *How do you usually handle conflicts regarding changes to your child's medical care plan?*

- *What might it look like to feel your child's fears of change rather than dismissing them?*

- *How might you live out your parental responsibility with greater courage, love, and understanding?*

Chapter Fifteen

Teach

Give a man a fish and you feed him for a day;
teach a man to fish and you feed him for a lifetime.
—ANCIENT PROVERB

Stepping into the kitchen, I see my son's diabetes supplies spread across the counter as he prepares his small overnight supply bag for a quick trip to New York with friends. He's catching the 2:20 p.m. train to Philadelphia where he will catch the Amtrak up to New York. Turning toward me, he inquires, "Mom, do we have any extra test strips in the house?"

"Did you check the pantry?" I ask, knowing that's the only place where extra strips might be.

"Yeah, but there weren't any in there."

He sees me eyeing the glucometer and the empty vial of test strips on the counter. "I didn't realize this vial of strips was empty when I left college for break. I didn't bring an extra bottle home with me."

He tests his blood sugar using his glucometer much less frequently now because he wears a continuous glucose monitor (CGM). But he still needs to check his blood sugar a few times a day with the glucometer—to calibrate the CGM and to make insulin-dosing decisions.

I look at him to see if he has a solution brewing in his mind. His eyes lock mine, yet he remains silent as he looks to me to guide us through this unexpected kink in his plan to go to New York.

"We'll have to call your pharmacy at school to have the prescription transferred here so we can fill it through insurance. By the way, when was the last time you ordered strips?" I ask.

"I picked some up last week," he answers. "They're the ones I left at school."

Great. That means we can't use our insurance. I offer to go to the pharmacy so he can continue getting organized for his trip. At CVS, the pharmacist quotes me the price for one box of strips without using insurance. I make a mental note to explain again to Austin exactly how insurance works. He may be an adult, but clearly I still have much to teach him about the cost of making mistakes.

Sensing my hesitation at the price, she adds, "You could also buy the CVS brand meter and one vial of our strips. That may be cheaper."

I make my way to the selection of meters, do a quick calculation, and sure enough, the store-brand meter and bottle of strips is the cheaper option. Paying for the items, I slip the bag into my purse and dash out to the car, pleased to have averted a real crisis.

I'm still pondering all I need to explain to my son more thoroughly—how insurance coverage works, how to buy diabetes supplies off insurance, my doubts about the reliability of this store-brand meter versus the meter he usually uses, and the importance of checking his supplies frequently, especially before a trip—when I pull into my garage. Walking in the back door, I shout to Austin that we should leave for the train in fifteen minutes.

Opening the refrigerator, I call up to him, "Did you pack your Lantus insulin?"

The next moment he's standing by my side. "No. Oh no. I think I left it at school too."

Lantus is his emergency insulin that he only uses if his insulin pump breaks; but we've learned the hard way always to be prepared for an emergency. He cannot go to New York without it. I shout a few commands at him, and we hastily get into the car with his overnight bag. Back to the CVS we go. Our stop will have to be quick or he will miss the train, so I call the pharmacy on the way.

"Hi, it's Bonnie O'Neil calling again…Yes, but it's for insulin this time…No, the prescription isn't in your files—you'll have to call Lewisburg Pharmacy for it…I'm so sorry, but can you expedite it? He's trying to catch a 2:20 p.m. train…Thanks, we'll be right there."

We tear into the store and approach the pharmacy counter. They promise us it will be ready in five more minutes. I look at my watch—we have eight minutes to spare. Five minutes pass. Six. Seven. Finally they hand us the bag containing the vial of life-saving liquid, and we make a mad dash for the car. We pull up to the train station with less than one minute to spare.

He gives me a quick hug before getting out of the car. Turning to look me in the eye, he beams that smile I love so well, the one that makes his eyes crinkle up into little slits of light.

"Thanks, Mom. Love you."

"I love you too, honey. Be safe. Have a good time. I'll see you tomorrow night."

The pounding in my heart subsides. My breathing slows to a normal rhythm. The crisis is behind us, but the importance of the moment isn't. There's so much still to teach my son, but today—in the midst of the crisis—is not the right time to sit at the teacher's desk and ask him to take notes. The lessons will come. Just not today.

As parents we are responsible for teaching our children about life. Whether they're toddlers or teenagers, or any age in between, it's common for them to engage with us in battles of the will as we try to teach them. Teaching them about nutrition, we tell them to eat their vegetables, and they clamp their mouths shut. Desiring for them to learn responsibility, we tell them to clean up their toys, and suddenly they are incapacitated with a terrible stomachache. As they grow, our conflicts may shift from their willful disobedience to their unintentional forgetfulness. Parenting would be so much easier if our children just did what we asked. But they don't, do they?

If we used arguing, berating, and yelling to settle conflicts when our children were young and willful, we may be inclined to continue that approach when they are distracted teenagers. *It's for their safety*, we rationalize. We're not simply trying to get them to eat their green beans. We understand that our child's carelessness could cost him dearly. And so, if we're not careful, we justify our reactions, saying that because it's for his safety, we have every right to raise our voice and criticize our child for not doing as we asked.

I don't want the management of my son's illness to dissolve into a battle of wills between us. Nor do I want him to perceive all my efforts at teaching as nothing more than a lifetime of nagging. If my goal is to win a particular battle—like what he chooses to eat for lunch, or how proactive he is at reviewing his blood sugar data, or whether he forgets some of his supplies at college—then I'm missing the point. My goal is to build a lifelong relationship with my son, built on love, respect, and trust. My goal is to raise a responsible adult who knows how to think for himself. When I make the success of his disease management my goal, I risk jeopardizing my relationship with my child.

When I make the success of his disease management my goal, I risk jeopardizing my relationship with my child.

I can be prone to reacting in the instant, afraid the teachable moment will slip away and I will have forever lost the opportunity to instruct my son. I'm not sure if I'm afraid that particular lesson will never present itself again, or if I'm afraid I'll forget to talk with him about it later. Perhaps I'm just impatient to see him learn everything now so I don't have to worry so much *later*. I can be too quick to open my mouth and share a nugget of wisdom, even if he's not in the right frame of mind to receive it and I'm not in the best mental state to deliver it. Just because the moment presents itself doesn't mean I have to teach a lesson right then and there. Gradually, over the space of many years, I'm coming to discover that what I say is not nearly as important as how or when I say it.

Losing my temper and venting a little steam just because I'm the mother doesn't make me the "winner." We both win when he learns to plan ahead. We win when we troubleshoot together what we could *both* do differently next time. We both win when I remember to praise him for the ninety-nine times he *has* remembered his supplies, making him feel good about his independence. We both lose when I yell enough to make him feel bad about himself. Even in the heat of the moment I have to keep in perspective that our parent-child relationship is far more precious than my relationship to him as his caregiver.

Caregiving requires us to keep the long view in mind, even when we would prefer to react in the moment. Exercising self-control is far more difficult than reacting for the sake of expediency, isn't it? When I exercise self-control in what I say and how I say it, I prioritize that which keeps our relationship healthy rather than those actions that shut it down. When I'm careful with my words, I earn the right to continue teaching my son.

When I'm careful with my words,
I earn the right to continue teaching my son.

Sometimes, like that day with the forgotten test strips and insulin, I exercise restraint and choose to save the teaching moment for another time when we're both calmer. An even greater challenge for me is identifying when it's better to say nothing at all than to repeat a lesson I know I've already taught him. It's hard to know which lessons should be taught in the moment, which ones should be set aside for another time, and which ones have already been taught enough. Not every lesson we have a mind to teach needs to be shared or shared again. I've discovered my son and I have a vastly different sense of how much time I spend teaching him. I think I share just enough, while he says sometimes diabetes is all we ever talk about.

I don't want this kind of conflict to define my relationship with my son. I want to practice loving him by looking for the right opportunities to teach him and recognizing when it's best to stay silent. My eagerness to share with him everything I've gleaned from studying his body's response to food, insulin, and exercise can overwhelm him and contribute to disease fatigue.

It helps when I remember the proverb: *Give a man a fish and you feed him for a day; teach a man to fish and you feed him for a lifetime.*

I have on many occasions given my son so many fish that they rotted in his hands. If I had given my son a fish as he was trying to catch that train, it would have slipped out of his hands and fallen onto the tracks as he boarded the train. When I practice patience and wait for the right opportunity to teach him, I actually feed my son for a lifetime by teaching him how to fish.

Heart to Heart

- *How do you typically react when your child doesn't manage his care as well as you would like?*

- *When you're at risk of engaging in a battle of wills, how could you begin to practice taking the long view rather than reacting for the sake of expediency?*

- *How has trying to be the "winner" in conflicts with your child hurt your relationship? What would it look like for you both to win?*

PART FOUR

All in the Family

Chapter Sixteen

A Separate Grief

In grief nothing "stays put." One keeps on emerging from a phase,
but it always recurs. Round and round. Everything repeats.
Am I going in circles, or dare I hope I am on a spiral?
—C.S. Lewis

My birthday was two days ago. I didn't feel much like celebrating. We're almost six weeks into our new life with T1D and things haven't really gotten any easier. Every day brings with it the same frustrations. Despite my best efforts, I can't seem to regulate my son's blood sugars. I get so depressed every time his glucometer reads too high or too low.

It seems like the disease is mine right now. I know it's Austin's illness, but he's too young to manage any of it by himself. His care falls 100 percent on my shoulders. I analyze his blood sugars and carbohydrates, calculating how much insulin to give or withhold. I draw up the insulin syringes. I test his blood sugar by finger prick. I plan what to take on every outing. I watch him like a hawk, and I worry.

Austin has been so good about it all, but I notice he is much more withdrawn now. Suddenly his thumb and blankie have become his constant companions. He seems happier when he's occupied with something fun to do outside the house. But every time we leave home it falls on me to restock our carry bag with his supplies—needles, insulin, glucose tabs, juice boxes, an assortment of snacks, alcohol wipes, a glucometer, test strips, and glucagon. Like a mother carrying an enormous diaper bag, I have to be ready for any eventuality.

I have no babysitters yet in our new town. I can't even imagine trusting someone enough to leave her in charge of managing a five-year-old with T1D. For now, every time I leave the house, we all go together. It's an added stress always trying to fit outings—even a trip to the grocery store—around the blood test-shot-meal-snack schedule. I've not just returned to the diaper bag days; it's like I'm reliving the schedule of a nursing mom.

Austin is learning to feel his low blood sugars. Despite my underlying state of anger that my son has T1D, I'm deeply thankful he feels his lows. Undetected lows are extremely dangerous, so it's critical that I quickly give him glucose to elevate his blood sugar when he's low. Like my sister, and many people with T1D, he describes his lows as feeling "shaky."

Most days I'm awakened by a hungry and shaky boy who needs food before I can even get a coffee. Most nights my sleep is disturbed by images of finger pricks, needles, and "what-if" scenarios. I worry about eating out and trying to correctly estimate carbohydrate values. When I think about Austin returning to school in the fall, my stomach ties in knots like necklaces tossed carelessly in a jewelry case. My need to be alert and "on" all day, coupled with night after night of restless sleep, leaves me in a state of emotional exhaustion.

I watch my husband and struggle to understand how he is processing any of this. "You have nothing to complain about," he rebuffs me when I grumble about our son getting T1D. "Even with Austin's diabetes, you still have it better than 99 percent of the world's population."

That may be true, but my mama heart has just broken into a million pieces, and today—and for the foreseeable future—I don't really care about the other 99 percent. Today all I see is my son and how his world has changed, and with it, mine. I'm in mourning for all that was lost, and my words take on the form of a lament, a wail, not a song of rejoicing.

"You don't understand," I holler at him. "You go off to work every day, and nothing in your world has changed. I can't leave the house for a minute. I can barely take a shower without someone coming to find me and telling me something is wrong. I can no longer eat a meal without doing math—estimating carbs and fat grams and calculating insulin to carbohydrate ratios. All day long I wonder, *What is he eating? Is he exercising? How are his blood sugars?* It's all I ever think about!"

"Well, everybody has something they think about every hour," he responds drily. "You're making this diagnosis all about you."

Rage boils inside me like an underground fault line preparing to erupt. I can't stand the sight of my husband right now. His complete detachment disgusts me. Is he a stoic that he shows no emotion? Good heavens, this is our son we're talking about! Shed a tear for your precious son, please. I want to shake him until he sees things from my point of view.

How can he move along from grief so quickly? Did he even grieve our son's loss of health and freedom? Does he even now understand all that has been lost? Perhaps not. He hasn't lived with the disease as I have with my sister. He wasn't raised with the specter of another T1D diagnosis as I was. He didn't lose a brother to this disease as I did.

I'm not asking him to jump right into anger like me. I wouldn't wish the state I'm in on my worst enemy. But what about some raw grief? How about a little denial? He has seemingly moved through all five stages of grief and settled right into acceptance without so much as batting an eyelash. Like a stone fortress, his emotions are impenetrable. He carries on, without any emotional fuss, as though his heart is fully intact.

His grief doesn't look like mine.

His grief doesn't look like mine.

Waves of anger roll over me as I realize we have traveled the same path together leading us to Austin's diagnosis, but on June 17 he turned one way while I turned the other. We are diverging faster now, as each one digs in, convinced of having found the right way to grieve.

Why won't he understand my perspective? Can't he see how things have changed for Austin? For me? I need to see his heart is also broken for our son. I need to know he's not coldhearted. I'm beginning to question the strength of his love for us. I don't understand what it means to receive this kind of diagnosis and *not* be brokenhearted.

Does he see me as weak because of my tears and complaints? Does he imagine a stronger woman would handle the shock and complexity of this disease better? I don't see myself as weak. Just exhausted. And realistic. I want what I cannot have. I want to go to the pawnshop, pay what's due, and get my former life back. But I can't have it. And so I cry and I grumble and I ask over and over again, *Why did this have to happen to our son?*

Does my husband want me to face all of life's challenges with a stiff upper lip because that's the way *he* makes it through a crisis? Does he need to look for the positive in every situation because the alternative is unthinkable to him? Is facing the reality of Austin's disease too much for him to handle, or does he truly think everything is okay?

I can handle not having his help with the added burdens of T1D. If I must care for our son day and night while he goes to work and while he sleeps, then so be it. I will do whatever it takes to keep our son as safe and healthy as possible. What I cannot handle is the accusation that my grief is out of place and somehow overexaggerated in comparison with the world's suffering. I simply cannot accept being judged for the way I grieve.

And yet I seem to so easily judge him for the way he grieves. Mutual acceptance is elusive in these early days and weeks. I need to know my husband will hold me through the pain, even if he doesn't feel the pain himself. And I suppose he needs to know I will hold him too.

Heart to Heart

- *How did you grieve when your child was diagnosed? How did your spouse grieve when your child was diagnosed?*

- *How have you as a couple handled the differences in your grieving processes?*

- *In what ways could you offer your spouse grace to grieve in his/her own way as you adjust to life with chronic illness?*

Chapter Seventeen

Resentment

Now that you don't have to be perfect, you can be good.
—JOHN STEINBECK

The robin swoops low from the holly tree, practically grazing my head that late-spring morning. It's the second clutch of eggs this robin couple has laid this year, and the parents are growing increasingly nervous at any movement we make, not just around the holly tree, but anytime we open our garage door or walk on the driveway. The mama robin and her proud, big-breasted mate take turns guarding the nest, hunting for food, feeding and caring for the babies, and swooping on the unsuspecting people who think the holly tree belongs to them.

I return to the house, newspaper in hand, choosing instead to watch the morning bird show from the theatre of my living room. In and out the parents fly, one by one making their more than one hundred daily foraging and feeding trips. I marvel that the energy with which they attend to their tasks appears no less significant in the evening hours than it does first thing in the morning. But more than their energy level impresses me; I am astounded at the cooperation, the togetherness, of this couple. They have a tremendous amount of work ahead of them each day, and yet they manage it all with an instinctive sense of purpose.

The contrast between the couple outside my window and the one living inside could not seem further apart.

Granted, the robins only have to keep up their frenetic pace for a few weeks while we have been living with the stress of chronic illness for several years. Still, I yearn for more of their sense of shared purpose.

It didn't take us long after our son's diagnosis to slip into our traditional roles—my husband as provider and I as caregiver. We had decided I would stay home to raise the children when they were young, so it made sense to continue in these roles now. But caring for a child with chronic illness requires the physical stamina of those robin parents, and I was having difficulty managing things all alone.

It's been close to four years, yet the nights never seem to get any easier. My son is growing, and that's a blessing. As he grows, his insulin needs increase, and it's extremely difficult to determine by how much. Counterbalancing those insulin increases is an increase in his activity— the inevitable sign that spring has returned. The more he exercises, the less insulin he needs. So, from one day to the next, it's nearly impossible to predict how much insulin is the right amount. I've been here before— last spring, and every prior spring and summer, have presented me with the same challenges and the same sleepless nights.

I head into the kitchen to clean up the breakfast dishes. I try to remember that my husband has to get up early and must function all day at work. Interrupted sleep is the last thing he needs. I remind myself that I *could* go back to bed once the children are at school, but I know I would never do that. It just feels wrong to me. Like it means I'm lazy, or not being truly myself, or, quite possibly, like the disease has won.

The nights when I have to check my son around the clock are particularly difficult. I set the alarm clock and clutch it to my chest, afraid I might not awaken if I return it to its usual place on the bedside table. The alarm rings in twenty-minute intervals, shocking me awake as with a blast of cold water while my husband lies peacefully asleep beside me.

During nights like these, nothing brings me to my senses faster than fear.

Or perhaps anger.

Fear and anger. My two companions since day one of the diagnosis. I had thought I would move beyond them as one moves through the stages of grief, arriving at acceptance, but here I am, several years later, still cycling in and out of fear and anger.

In the dark hours of sleep interruption, I don't know what makes me angrier—that he won't get up during the night or that I don't trust him to actually test our son's blood sugar. I've witnessed too many times when he was "on duty" that he either didn't wake up from the alarm, or he got up, walked to the other room, and promptly got back into bed without testing our son.

I'm seething now at the knowledge that I can't trust my husband with the alarm and nearly drop a glass in the sink. I tell myself that if he would do just one of the nighttime checks, I could push through my exhaustion. And if I could push through my exhaustion, then perhaps I could suppress the resentment growing in my heart.

If I'm honest, my list of resentments is growing by the week. With the self-righteousness of one who is clearly still licking her open wounds, I stand mighty and proud, judge and jury, and pass my judgments.

It's not just the nights; he doesn't help enough during the waking hours either. All the burden of caregiving falls on me.

He really hasn't learned much about this disease—certainly not enough to make any decisions related to our son's care. All the burden of decision-making falls on me.

He never mourned for our son's losses as I did. All the burden of loving and empathizing falls on me.

I drop my gavel. *Guilty as charged.*

I steep in my resentment toward him. How could he leave me feeling so *abandoned*? My resentment festers like a wound gone septic.

My mind turns the word over a few more times—*abandoned*—as I realize it's most likely the same judgment my husband passes down on me. He tells me I've lost perspective, that I place too much focus on the disease, and that I'm ignoring him as I thrust all my emotional energy on our son. I dismiss him as being cold-hearted, un-feeling, and unrealistic about the demands of the disease.

A seemingly insurmountable chasm has developed between us, made wider by the force of the selfish words that churn within our tempestuous minds and flow from our mouths. Antagonism grows between us at the smallest difference of opinion related to our son's care. We're hostile as we defend our expectations of one another.

Resentment grows like a snowball rolling ever faster and growing exponentially larger with every 360-degree turn until finally it blocks the way forward. We are trapped. I'm frozen on one side, my spouse on the other. I begin to understand why some couples don't survive these kinds of diagnoses, and I'm determined not to be one of them.

Resentment breeds in the gap between my expectation of my spouse's actions and the reality of how he chooses to act. I provide fertile soil for resentment to grow when I refuse to allow his responses to painful or stressful situations to be different from mine. My disappointment in him confirms to me that my approach to raising a child with chronic illness is the only correct and acceptable one.

But what if he's right? What if I've abandoned him too?

I know it's my fear for our son's well-being that drives me to go it alone. My mama need to protect him propels me to get up in the night when necessary, to count every carbohydrate he puts in his mouth, to insist the insulin calculations fall on my shoulders. My fear whispers to me not to trust anyone else with my son's care.

As if a quiet voice of reason whispers truth to me, I see it—my husband is also afraid. He's afraid he won't be able to manage our son's care as well as I do. He's afraid he won't be able to function the next day at work if he's exhausted, and so he fears for his ability to provide for us. He's afraid of making a mistake that could cost our son his life.

Maybe my way *is* the better way, maybe his is. But maybe, just maybe, each of us is doing the best we can, given our temperaments, our abilities, and the established patterns within our family unit. Perhaps the real issue is not who is right and who is wrong, but rather how willing I am to forgive my spouse for not living up to my expectations.

We develop the practice of resentment by harboring a habit of unforgiveness. Unforgiveness sits like burning acid in the gut. It will continue to destroy us until we purge ourselves of it.

> *We develop the practice of resentment*
> *by harboring a habit of unforgiveness.*

Forgiveness is never easy, but it's the only remedy to cure resentment. When I forgive, I release the stranglehold that my need to be right has over me. Forgiveness is a choice, a decision made over and over again to give up any claim of requital or restitution. Forgiveness is the greatest model of selfless love because it requires nothing less than the laying down of my rights to get my own way.

When I forgive, I learn how to accept the consequences of someone else's actions even if those consequences are painful to me. When I choose to forgive rather than remain locked in patterns of bitterness and resentment, I choose to live in the freedom that comes when I accept things I cannot change. American theologian Reinhold Niebuhr expresses this concept well in his famous prayer:

God grant me the serenity to accept the things I cannot change,
Courage to change the things I can,
And wisdom to know the difference.

Forgiveness is needed in the chasm between disappointment and acceptance of what is and must be practiced repeatedly until disappointment gives way to acceptance.

Forgiveness is needed in the chasm
between disappointment and acceptance
of what is and must be practiced repeatedly
until disappointment gives way to acceptance.

The invitation to forgive rises before me like a beacon of light, illuminating enough of the path before me that I can make a few tentative steps in its direction. I have a long way to go before I can offer generous helpings of grace and forgiveness to my husband on a regular basis, but I think I am now at least oriented on the right path. Forgiveness, it turns out, is a vital component of putting love into action.

Heart to Heart

- *In what ways have resentment and bitterness seeped into your relationship with your spouse?*

- *How have feelings of abandonment factored into your feelings of resentment?*

- *What might forgiveness look like for you? What direction will you take as you stand at the crossroads of resentment and forgiveness?*

Chapter Eighteen

Am I Next?

If you can stand the upsetting energy, you may be allowed to watch
while dark and light come back into balance.
—Barbara Brown Taylor

Growing up with two siblings with T1D, my greatest fear was that I would get the family disease. My mother also feared for Betsy and me. After Barb's diagnosis, every few months my mother would hand Betsy and me a little gray box of urine test strips and ask us to check if we had diabetes.

"Clip off a strip and pee on it," she instructed us. "Wait thirty seconds and compare it to the color chart on the side panel. If it changes color, bring it to me right away. Otherwise, throw it away."

I would dutifully do as she instructed me, careful to count the full thirty seconds before comparing my wet strip to the color-coded chart. I held my breath just a little bit as I counted down those thirty seconds. My strips never changed color, nor did Betsy's, but the memory of fear imprinted on our minds.

I understand the fear of getting a sibling's disease because I was afraid of getting T1D my entire childhood and well into adulthood.

My other two children, like me, also grew up afraid of getting T1D. Like me, they also harbored an unspoken anxiety that they would die at age eight, the age of my brother's death. My children were not the only ones in my family to experience fear of getting diabetes. All their cousins on my side of the family shared this similar concern. When my niece's two-month-old son was diagnosed with retinoblastoma, a cancer of the eye, she said to her mother, Betsy, "I always thought it would be diabetes. I never thought one of my kids would get cancer, just diabetes."

When chronic illness afflicts a young person, other family members often respond with a heightened experience of fear of illness. Parents and siblings alike have had their eyes opened to potential dangers they didn't worry about before. With a sibling's diagnosis, a seemingly safe world can suddenly appear threatening and foreboding. Even if your child was born with his condition, his siblings may fear being afflicted with a different disorder that develops after birth. Your other children may not speak openly of it, but fear has more than likely sidled up to them and seeped under their skin.

Fear can be subtle, simmering below the surface like a teakettle on a low boil. Or it might loom large, incapacitating our children from moving forward. As parents, our role is to understand the place fear occupies in our children's lives and help them find ways of addressing it. It may help for them to speak with a counselor if their fear is overwhelming or if they are unwilling to speak with us about it. Often though, if we create safe spaces for them to share honestly, they will open up with us about their fears.

We might begin by sharing a story with our children of how fear gripped us. This probably won't diminish their own fear, but it invites them to express their anxiety to us, trusting we won't deny or dismiss what they feel. If we want to encourage our children to share their most private emotions with us, we begin by acknowledging their fear. We don't want to shut them down by saying their anxiety is unwarranted.

Our children may be too young to fully understand their fear; they just know they're afraid. Sharing with our little ones that sometimes we're afraid too may coax them to reveal just a little more. Our teenage children may feel ashamed of their fear, thinking they need to be brave, so they suppress their feelings and remain silent. Our teenagers, especially, need a safe place to share the worries they carry.

When we attend carefully to our children's fears, we hold their fear for them, exposing it to the light so they can identify it and name it. The first step to overcoming fear is naming it for what it is. Only then can we begin to understand its power in our life. Attending to fear requires courage and a willingness to sit with our children in the uncertainty as we help them wrestle through their fear to a place of hope.

It may get loud—as they cry out their fears. It may remain deafeningly silent—as we search to no avail for words of comfort. It will rip our hearts—as we see the depths of our child's anxiety and our inability to make it all right. But fear exposed is always better than fear left buried. When left untended, fear stiffens us, like blood run cold, until rigor mortis prevents us from living fully alive. Fear exposed to the light, even if messy and painful, reminds us all hope is not lost.

Fear exposed to the light, even if messy and painful, reminds us all hope is not lost.

In their fear, I seek to help them remember hope. I know what they cannot yet know—that hope is stronger than despair. And love is stronger than fear.

Heart to Heart

- *How have you explored with your other children the fear they carry of getting their sibling's disease?*

- *How do you handle your own fears of a second diagnosis within your family?*

- *In what ways could you help your children move through fear to a place of hope and love?*

Chapter Nineteen

Sibling Rivalry

I sustain myself with the love of family.
—MAYA ANGELOU

I dreaded Austin's first Halloween. A day dedicated to gorging on candy is a recipe for disaster for a six-year-old boy without a functioning pancreas. I prepared him in advance that Halloween would be different that year and every year to come. I wouldn't be able to draw up a syringe of insulin on our dark street, so he wouldn't be able to enjoy his candy until we returned home. Then he could eat one or two pieces from his Halloween bag before going to bed.

The night went better than I expected. His blood sugar dropped while we were trick-or-treating, so he got to eat a piece of candy after all—to elevate his blood sugar while he ran from house to house. After eating another piece when we got home, he placed his bright orange plastic pumpkin container with the black carry strap on the kitchen counter. Every day for the next month he would dig through it for a piece of candy, until he forgot all about Halloween and I threw the rest of the candy away.

This is his second Halloween with T1D. Austin is dressed up as a Philadelphia Phillies baseball player. Many of the neighborhood children and some of their parents have gathered next door for a quick pizza dinner before the children scatter to canvass the street. Alexander joins the older children while I stay close to Austin and Alicia as we make our way through the neighborhood together. Up to the cul-de-sac and back down to the other end of our street we roam until we ring all thirty-seven doorbells, cheerfully exclaiming, "Trick or treat!"

I'm deeply moved by the thoughtfulness of many of my neighbors. Instead of offering my son candy, they prepared goody bags of toys and tchotchkes for him. One neighbor's gift bag was so big it was nearly half Austin's size. It was filled with balls and board games, activity books and books to read. It even included a backyard paddleball set. I don't think I've ever experienced this kind of thoughtfulness and generosity before. I thank each of them, breathing a sigh of relief that, because of their kindness, Halloween won't be so bad for my son after all.

It's late by the time the children finish digging through their loot, sorting their candy by favorites and setting aside anything they want to contribute to our candy bowl for the late-night trick-or-treaters. We all head upstairs together, yawning as we go. I help Alicia out of her unicorn costume and into her pajamas as the boys get themselves ready for bed. One child tucked in. Two more to go.

Heading first to Austin's room, I open his door and step inside. Thankfully, he's already under the covers. *Good, bedtime will be easy tonight.* As I approach his bed, I notice he's lying on his side, his face turned away from me.

"Wasn't that a fun Halloween?" I ask as I sit on the bed next to him.

In the dark with his back to me, he lets out a sniffle. Before he says a word, I know he's crying. "Why does everyone else get to have as much candy as they want? I want to eat candy like everyone else can. I didn't even get much candy this year; I just got toys."

I'm stunned. This wasn't what I was expecting to hear from him. I thought he would be as delighted by the gifts as I was. Instead, they made him feel singled out. Different. Reminded that he can no longer eat candy with abandon. But still, would he really prefer to get a lot of candy that he can't eat than get an assortment of toys he could enjoy over and over again for many months to come?

"What do you mean?" I ask him cautiously. "I thought it was so kind of our neighbors to give you those nice gifts instead of candy. Don't you think it was nice of them?"

"I guess," he whispers. "But I just want to be able to eat candy like everyone else. It's not fair!"

Ahh, the dreaded *it's not fair* remark. This doesn't feel like the right time to launch into a lesson on fairness in our broken world. That's a critical lesson for all parents to teach their children, especially if they have a child with chronic illness. But Halloween night, when everyone is already exhausted, just doesn't seem like the right time.

And so I make a few more attempts to remind my son of our friends' kindness. I tell him he is loved and cherished, and he has a neighborhood full of friends standing by his side. Not convinced I've helped cheer him up, I'm nevertheless ready to end tonight's tuck-in. I pray with him, kiss him gently goodnight, and slip out of his room. Still surprised by how Austin responded to the generosity of our friends, I open Alexander's door for the final tuck-in of the evening. I begin to speak as I make my way to sit on his bed.

"What a nice Halloween, wasn't it?"

Without paying any attention to my question, my son shoots back, "Why does Austin always get all the toys and gifts? All I get on Halloween is candy, and he got all kinds of presents. It's not fair!"

Are you kidding me? I want to shout at him! I muster an ounce of self-control before opening my mouth. "Sweetie, Austin can't eat candy like you and your sister can. Our neighbors were very kind to think about that and to get some special things for him so he wouldn't feel left out. Can't you see they were just being thoughtful?"

"Yeah, but he always gets everything."

I pause before responding. "Sometimes he may get an extra toy or a book, but he experiences a lot of hard things every day because of his diabetes. I don't think you want to start comparing your life to his on a basis of what's fair. Our neighbors love you as much as they love Austin, and so do I."

I really don't want to get into a conversation about fairness with my nine-year-old either, so I pray quickly with him, kiss him goodnight, and quietly close the door behind me. Standing in the hallway, emotionally and physically drained, I wonder how the three of us could have perceived such a beautiful night in three completely different ways.

Raised on the companion ideals of the Declaration of Independence, which asserts *all men are created equal*, and the Pledge of Allegiance, which ends with a promise of *liberty and justice for all*, American children pay particular attention to issues of fairness in their own lives. While some children learn at a young age that their particular demographic doesn't benefit from the same level of freedom or prosperity as another demographic may, they expect to find equity and justice within their own tight community. Grant one child in a family or classroom a privilege over another child and you are sure to hear the familiar cry: *that's not fair!*

We expect fairness to be woven into the fabric of our family life. And when the family landscape doesn't appear to be 100 percent equitable, sibling rivalry results. All families experience some form of sibling rivalry. Families that live with chronic illness are certainly no exception.

Children living with chronic illness learn all too early that life isn't fair. They examine their lives compared to those of their siblings and friends and find their lives coming up short. Their daily lives are more challenging, and their futures are filled with more uncertainty. It's common for children with chronic illness to experience jealousy toward their siblings and friends.

Children living with chronic illness learn all too early that life isn't fair.

Interestingly, our children living with chronic illness are not the only ones to experience sibling rivalry. Their siblings—who have also discovered early that life isn't fair—are also susceptible to feelings of jealousy toward their sibling with chronic illness. Our other children can perceive the extra time and attention we give to their sibling as our parental preference for that child. In a child's mind, time plus attention equals love. Using this equation to define love sets up children in families with chronic illness to experience sibling rivalry.

Familiar lies repeat within the heart and mind of a child experiencing sibling rivalry like a soundtrack on a continuous loop. *My parents pay more attention to her than they do to me. They don't love me as much as they love him. My parents don't even see me anymore; they only have eyes for my sibling. I have to work harder to win their love.* Our children may verbalize some of this inner conflict with us, but often, like their fear of getting the disease, they keep these thoughts locked inside. When we witness our child increasingly criticizing their sibling for no obvious reason, or criticizing us for the amount of time we spend with their sibling, we should be on the lookout for sibling rivalry.

Alicia was too young when Austin was diagnosed to have a sense for how our life had changed. Alexander, on the other hand, was keenly aware of what had changed and how marginalized he felt as a result. In those early months he began criticizing his brother, picking on him, and complaining about unimportant things. Initially I pushed back,

Chapter Twenty

Three Musketeers

I have simply tried to do what seemed best each day, as each day came.
—Abraham Lincoln

It's Pizza Night at Jack's house when I pick up Austin from an afternoon playing with his best friends, Jack and Chris. They have been Austin's dearest friends since we moved to Pennsylvania three years ago. Their mothers, Jeanne and Patti, have always been exceedingly kind to Austin and to me.

From the earliest days of our sons' friendship, they asked me thoughtful questions, genuinely interested in learning everything they needed to keep Austin safe while he was at their homes. They stocked their pantries with juice boxes and mini bags of pretzels and Goldfish to give him when his blood sugar dropped too low. They fostered close relationships with my son so he felt comfortable speaking to them when he didn't feel well. They were the surrogate moms who advocated on his behalf to coaches, umpires, and referees if I was ever running late to a game. In these two homes Austin had his first, long-awaited sleepovers, made possible because my friends had created safe environments for my son. They were even willing to get up in the night for a blood sugar test if needed. Every mom with a child with chronic illness needs friends like these.

The scent of pizza hangs in the air as I step into the kitchen. I'll never understand how the smell of three simple ingredients—bread, cheese, and sauce—when combined together and baked in a brick oven can create such pure magic. The aroma itself tells me to slow down; a time of relaxation and pleasure awaits us.

My dinner, on the other hand—which as yet lives only in my mind— is grilled chicken, roasted vegetables, and rice. Nothing about it speaks of relaxation and pleasure. It's a sensible meal, comprised of the three USDA recommended components of protein, vegetable, and starch. It will take me close to an hour to wash, chop, roast, marinate, grill, boil, and serve my family this meal. Calling for pizza and selecting the at-home delivery option sounds so much more appealing to me right now.

How I long to cancel my family dinner plans, ring up the pizza shop from my friend's kitchen, and have a hot, steaming pizza delivered to us minutes after we arrive home tonight. This vision of a simplified evening rises before my eyes, and I find myself wanting this pizza like a teenage girl desperate to have the latest fashion fad. I'm exhausted from another series of sleepless nights testing blood sugars. I yearn to exchange my hour preparing a healthy meal with a phone call promising me that relaxation and pleasure will penetrate the walls of my hearth and heart.

Occasionally we do get pizza for dinner, usually on a Friday, because I want to celebrate making it through another week of work and school. Somehow pizza feels like a treat to me, mostly because I don't have to cook, but also because the children are delighted to discover Pizza Night has replaced our sensible meal. But the magic quickly dissipates when Austin's blood sugars begin their eight-hour excursion of dips and surges as his body tries to metabolize the excessive fat and carbohydrate contained in two slices of cheese pizza. It may smell like a gift from the gods, but I can assure you, pizza is no gift to the body. No matter how many ways I try to modify his insulin flow when he eats food like pizza, cheesesteak, Chinese food, and most restaurant meals, I can't seem to find the right dose of insulin at the right timing to counterbalance the effect of his rising blood sugar. More and more I'm discovering that while Pizza Night begins as a treat for the family, it ends up meaning a sleepless night for me.

Standing in my friend's kitchen, I push back feelings of envy as Austin ties his shoes and gathers his belongings. I have reached a certain level of acceptance with this disease, but occasional jealousy still catches me off-guard like a thief in the night coming to steal my joy. I suppose I could have done things differently in our family from the earliest days post-diagnosis. I could have restricted Austin's diet while the rest of us carried on eating foods that were too much for his body to handle. But that approach didn't hold much appeal for me. I want him to feel even more comfortable in his own home than he does in the homes of his two dear friends. I don't want mealtimes to draw any more attention to the differences between him and his siblings. Those differences are evident enough as we tend to the management of his blood sugars. If he can't safely eat pizza, we'll all eat less pizza.

Chronic illness isolates. As a caregiver, I have felt isolated from my friends, as if a line of demarcation has been drawn between us. I imagine you've felt the same sense of exclusion. Although our friends try to understand, they don't bear the continual weight of the burden we carry. We stand alone on the side designated for those with a child with chronic illness, while they stand together on the other side. In the gap between us, isolation brews.

We know isolation, but our children know it far more intimately than we ever will. Every day your child's disease identifies him as *different* from his peers. None of us enjoys being singled out, unless perhaps to accept an award or be praised. But our children with chronic illness are singled out all the time. At school they are the *frequent flyers* in the nurse's office. In the classroom they may be accompanied by an aide or have to step out of the classroom for additional support. School singles out children who are different.

Other environments pose additional challenges to the child with special needs. Before my son began using an insulin pump, meals at restaurants always elicited raised eyebrows from fellow diners. I would feel multiple pairs of eyes boring into us when I drew up his insulin to inject him at the table. Going through airport security, my son can never remain anonymous. He must remove his insulin pump, hand it to a TSA agent, and carefully explain what it is and why it can't go through security. How many times in his young life has my son wanted to crawl under the table and disappear?

Chronic illness differentiates our children not just from friends and strangers, but also from their siblings. I couldn't control how people in the outside environment treated my son, but I desperately wanted him to feel as normal as possible in his home. I don't know if my efforts succeeded, but I tried to blur that line of distinction as much as possible.

In his book *The Three Musketeers*, Alexandre Dumas made famous the line "One for all, and all for one!" As we began navigating life with chronic illness, this seemed a fitting motto for us to adopt as well. My heart began to settle into one new priority—to preserve unity and love within our family as best as possible.

---

*My heart began to settle into one new priority—
to preserve unity and love within our family
as best as possible.*

Fully embracing love and unity are lofty goals for any family. Imagine the challenge for a family living with chronic illness. How can we possibly live united when the particular needs of one of our children clearly differentiate him from the rest of the family? Is it even possible to navigate the tension between meeting the needs of one child and the desires of the others?

I wrestled with these issues in the early years, intent on discovering workable solutions to these hard questions. I wondered if my love was expansive enough to commit to the hard work of nurturing unity within my family despite these challenges. Every family is unique, so the particular practices we adopt to foster unity will vary among us. In my family, because of Austin's T1D, our central issue revolved around food choices. Would I restructure only Austin's meals, or would we all adjust?

I approached this question from the standpoint of my overarching vision regarding family meals. My husband and I had lived in France several times and had adopted their national love for *the table*. While breakfast and lunch were simpler undertakings, dinner always meant a time to linger around a shared meal. The food was as delicious and fresh as the conversation was honest and open. A French dinner is an opportunity to celebrate family seven days a week, fifty-two weeks a year.

I carried this tradition back with me after we left Paris when Alexander was less than a year old. It shaped how I thought about food and how I envisioned our family dinners would be. When Austin was diagnosed with a disease so impacted by food choices, I had to think more carefully about what we ate. I knew I wanted to hold onto our cherished shared family dinners, so that meant we all had to eat foods that were healthy choices for Austin. I stopped making some meals, or made them less frequently, because they would wreak havoc on his blood sugars. Fresh vegetables occupied an increasingly larger portion on our dinner plates. Shortcuts in the kitchen weren't possible, not if I really wanted to focus on healthy nutrition.

I also had to be mindful of when we ate. Because insulin takes three hours to work through the human body, I needed to be sure we ate early enough that most of his insulin had finished working by the time he went to bed. Nights when the kids had sports practices or games were especially difficult. I had to get creative—preparing a late afternoon dinner—so we could eat together before an early evening activity. With a little advance planning, I never had to rely on fast food, and we somehow always managed to eat together.

In addition to thinking more intentionally about food, I had to develop some guiding principles regarding family activities. Chronic illness imposes time and logistics constraints on us, especially when our children are very young. I began thinking about after-school activities and summer camps like I thought about food. We would live united.

In the early years carpooling wasn't an option because I had to stay with Austin during his activities. So we would all pile in the car and go together. If I wasn't comfortable sending Austin to a summer day camp, then I wouldn't send the other two either. I didn't want to promote opportunities for jealousy to fester within the family. In those years, we spent a lot of time hanging out together as a family—entertaining ourselves during Austin's sports practices and taking summer excursions to the zoo, the aquarium, the pool, a park, the library, or Old City Philadelphia.

My two main issues—food and activities—might be very different from yours. Perhaps the way I approached meals and activities isn't appealing to you or doesn't fit with your family's rhythm. We each have to find the balance that works for our own family. One size definitely does not fit all. But you will need a philosophy for approaching how you fit chronic illness into the daily life of your family. My objective was to help my son see a level playing field within the security of his own home. I know the playing field wasn't truly level. And so did he. His daily regimen was reminder enough of that. But hopefully he felt he was given the same opportunities as his siblings.

I have observed a particular closeness between my children over the years, and a remarkable lack of fighting throughout their childhood. Maybe it had something to do with the intentional time we spent together and the importance I placed on equity in the home. Maybe it was pure grace, a tender gift to us because of the challenges our family has endured. Maybe it was both. Looking back over the long and sometimes bumpy road behind me, I see how the intention to live *one for all, and all for one* has served us well.

Heart to Heart

- *How has chronic illness isolated your child from her peers? Her siblings?*

- *What aspects of your home life draw attention to the differences between your child with chronic illness and the rest of the family?*

- *What changes might you make to bridge the gap so your child doesn't feel so different?*

Chapter Twenty-One

Get Out There!

Life moves pretty fast. If you don't stop and look around once in a while, you could miss it.
—Ferris Bueller

Today is the day. The day we finally move to London with our family. We had danced around the idea of relocating there for close to three years. When my husband, Jon, was first offered the position to run his company's European operation, Austin's diabetes was still quite new. We had only lived in Pennsylvania for about a year, and I frankly couldn't envision moving again so soon. I had moved enough before and had lived overseas a couple of times, so I understood how medical systems differed from one country to the next. I was still learning so much about T1D; I had no capacity to mine the inner workings of the UK's National Health Service (NHS).

We said *no* to that first offer because I was tired and afraid. But when the offer was presented again two years later, we had just enough courage to consider accepting it. Pretty quickly we realized we desperately wanted to live in Europe again, and we wanted our children to experience living as expatriates with us. *It could be the adventure of a lifetime*, we thought.

I nervously zip up the last of the carry-on bags, the one containing all of Austin's diabetes supplies. I had ordered a three-month supply—the most I could purchase using our insurance—to give myself time once in the UK to find a doctor, get prescriptions, and figure out our insurance with the NHS. Most of the belongings we were taking to London had already left by sea container a few weeks before. I had everything organized so that even if there were a delay in Customs, we had enough in our ten suitcases and five carry-on bags to tide us over for several weeks.

The most important bag is this one containing Austin's diabetes supplies. They fill the entire roll-aboard bag. I pause to reflect that just three days ago, we didn't even know if we would be allowed to take *any* carry-on luggage, let alone one containing needles and lancing devices and 100 ml of insulin.

On August 10, 2006, one week before our scheduled move to London, a plot to blow up transatlantic airliners was discovered, and twenty-four people were brought into custody in the UK. Immediate restrictions were placed on all liquids and gels on all airplanes. Initially, *no liquids and no hand luggage* were allowed on any flights going in and out of the UK and the US. The UK raised its threat level to "critical," meaning an attack was expected imminently. John Reid, British Home Secretary, said, "Britain is facing its most sustained period of serious threat since the end of the second World War."[6]

I watched the news like a mama bird protecting her nest from a scavenger hawk. Every few hours I refreshed the British Airways alert page, desperate to discover if things had moved in our favor. After a few days the restrictions started to shift. Small handheld bags were allowed, but still no liquids. Then just a few milliliters of liquid were permitted,

6   "Mass murder terror plot uncovered," The Guardian, Aug. 10, 2006, www.google.com/amp/s/amp.theguardian.com/world/2006/aug/10/terrorism.politics.

certainly not enough for the minimum two bottles of insulin needed for even a weekend trip. No mention was made of any exceptions for lifesaving medication. I needed to find another way to get Austin's supplies over to London.

FedEx. I'll ship them by FedEx, I concluded, half confident of my plan. Hurriedly I took the supplies out of the small suitcase they were already packed in, grabbed the insulin from the refrigerator, placed everything in a cardboard box, and made my way to the local FedEx store.

Placing the box of supplies on the counter, I explained my predicament. "We're moving to London in four days, and if the ban on hand luggage doesn't change, I won't be able to take my son's diabetes supplies with us. Can you help us? Can you ship these supplies?"

"Yes, we should be able to ship those for you. What exactly is in your box there?" the man asks me.

"Well, it's insulin syringes, insulin pump supplies, an extra pump, lancets, an extra glucometer, test strips, glucagon, and insulin." I look at him hard, hopeful for the first time in days that maybe, just maybe, we have a solution.

He confers with a colleague and returns, smiling. "Yes, we can ship this for you. I can't guarantee exactly when you'll get it because it will have to go through Customs. Sometimes things sit on the docks for quite a while before being shipped out on the other end. Oh, by the way, there's nothing in here that could be damaged by sitting in the sun on a hot dock, is there?"

With that one question, my heart drops into my toes. "Yes. All of it. None of it should sit in the sun for a long time, especially not the insulin."

"I'm sorry, ma'am," he says to me, "I really am. But we can't assume the risk of shipping something that could be damaged by sitting on a dock for a few weeks. You'll have to find another way."

I tried begging him, but it was no use. I gathered my large box in my arms, left the store, slipped into my hot car, and cried. I had only been in the store for twenty minutes and my car already felt like an oven. Of course I couldn't ship my son's supplies by FedEx in the depths of August heat. Admitting defeat, I drove home slowly, questioning our decision to uproot our family, leave the safety of our country and medical system, and expose our children to such risk.

For three more days we watched the news and hoped the restrictions would lift. Today I tore off the last calendar page marking that our time in Pennsylvania has come to an end. Just yesterday we learned we were each allowed one traditional-sized carry-on bag. The ban on liquids still stands. In this heightened security environment, I can't imagine any TSA inspector allowing our bag of sharp objects and liquid to pass through security. In my mind, I see it all going in the trash and our little family of five being stopped for questioning. I finish zipping the bag and add it to the other fourteen sitting by our front door, awaiting the limo to take us to an uncertain future.

Raising a child with chronic illness requires enormous courage. It's not for the faint of heart. Yet there's no advance training before the diagnosis comes and no opportunity to flex your courage muscles in advance. Overnight, the life we understand and think we are controlling becomes complicated and uncertain. Eventually we adjust to our new normal. But sometimes in the adjustment we find ourselves more risk-averse than we were pre-diagnosis.

When our world shifts as dramatically as it does when chronic illness strikes, we naturally experience an increased desire to protect the ones we love. Like a batter in an 0-2 count, we close in to protect. Self-protection can take many forms. We may find ourselves reducing the number of family outings we take because it's more complicated to travel now. Opportunities that would have excited us in the past we may now consider too risky. We may even conclude it's too dangerous to have any more children. Often we simply close ourselves off to joy, having discovered firsthand how uncertain life can be. Over time the weight of chronic illness can lead us to give up hope as we conclude, "I have to play it safe. I can't risk another heartbreak."

The temptation toward self-protection can sneak up on us unawares, and if we aren't on the lookout for it, we might close ourselves off to life's opportunities for fear of the unknown. With our eye always on our child's illness, we can tend to filter every major decision, and many insignificant ones, through the lens of the disease. When we analyze our decisions in this way, all we see are the constraints—real and imagined—caused by our child's illness.

With our eye always on our child's illness, we can tend to filter every major decision, and many insignificant ones, through the lens of the disease.

There are real constraints when raising a child with T1D. I have to be careful about the food I give my son, making certain to know the nutritional information. I have to carry supplies with us at all times. I need to be certain we have access to excellent medical care. I've discovered, however, that many constraints are simply of my own perception and are not necessarily shared by other T1D parents. These constraints are based on my fears or my fatigue. If I'm honest, often I'm simply unwilling to accept any new element of risk.

Raising a family with a chronically ill child is most likely harder than you anticipated when you signed up for Parenting 101. You may be scared about what the future holds. I was too. Many days, I still worry about my son's future. As real as that fear is, we can't let it block us from living a full life. We need courage to keep moving forward into an unknowable future.

When my family was first offered the opportunity to live overseas, all I could think about was how I would manage Austin's diabetes in a country whose medical system I didn't quite understand. I couldn't see the unique opportunity set before us; all I could see were the risks related to my son's disease. We let go of that first chance to move to London out of my fear of the unknown. Admittedly, I was still dealing with extreme exhaustion and stress in that first year post-diagnosis and post-relocation to Pennsylvania. But mostly I was on an illusory quest for safety.

Evaluating life only through the eyes of an illness can lead us to make decisions to "sit things out" without even considering the benefits to everyone else in the family. As parents, our responsibility is to take into consideration the needs of the entire family, not just the impact of a decision on the child with chronic illness. When we remove the telephoto lens we so often use to evaluate our child's health, in exchange for a wide-angle lens that captures the needs of the whole family, we begin to see things more clearly.

With new eyes, I could see it was the right decision for my husband's career. I realized it would be a tremendous opportunity for all my children to discover new things about themselves and the world. And I remembered how much I had loved living in Paris and had always dreamed of living abroad again with my family. With a mind finally open to the possibilities, I stepped out in courage. *If I gave birth in France*, I mused, *of course I can figure out how to manage T1D in England.*

Acting from a place of courage doesn't mean our problems go away, it just means we've learned to take action despite our fears.

Acting from a place of courage doesn't mean our problems go away, it just means we've learned to take action despite our fears. There's a lot of life ahead for your family. This illness is a part of your story, but it doesn't have to be the central plot line. You may have times of doubt and fear, times when you want to eliminate all possible risk and simplify so much that you forget to live. Can I encourage you not to do that? The world needs what you and your family can uniquely contribute to it. Don't give up. Get out there!

Our ten large bags move along the conveyor belt, beckoning us to come find them again once we arrive in London's Heathrow Airport. One final hurdle remains—the security checks of our five carry-on bags, including the one with over a hundred sharp needles and far more liquid than we are authorized to carry.

We approach the makeshift TSA security table as a family. I tell everyone to stay calm and above all to present themselves as quiet, respectful children. I'm hoping we can slide through without much notice. The tall man with the dark skin and kind eyes informs us every one of the five bags will be individually inspected. *Can he hear my heart pounding from across the table*, I wonder?

The first four bags are opened and inspected and returned to us. The last bag is Austin's. I had placed it last, hoping the agent would wave us on after finding four clean bags. No such luck. As the agent unzips Austin's bag, I speak the words I have rehearsed for just this moment. "I'm traveling with my son who has type 1 diabetes. We are moving to London. These are his diabetes supplies."

He looks up at me and over to Austin. "Is this your son?" he asks kindly.

"Yes, sir," I reply quietly and respectfully.

He opens the bag and eyes the first object lying on top of all the supplies—my husband's big black Bible. He had placed it there at the last minute because there was no room for it in his large suitcase. The agent looks up at us. "Ahh, God's Word. An important book to read."

"Yes, sir," my husband replies. "I try to read it every day."

"So do I, young man. So do I." He carefully zips the bag and hands it back to us. "Enjoy your time in England, and be well."

Just like that, our worries about needles and excess liquid evaporate and we are off on the adventure of a lifetime. Sometimes I wonder what our life would have been like if I had said yes the first time we were offered to move to London. Our two years there gave us the priceless gift of growing closer as a family. Living in a small apartment, walking to and from school together, learning how to live in a city in a foreign country, we grew to depend on one another like we never had before. The world opened up to us when we chose to live courageously despite chronic illness. I can't imagine what our lives would have been like if I had said *no* the second time.

Heart to Heart

- *In what ways have you begun to make family decisions based solely on the constraints of your child's condition? If you're honest, are these constraints real or imagined?*

- *How has your child's chronic illness reduced your willingness for risk and increased your need for safety in your family life?*

- *What steps might you take today to live more courageously, with a heart open to more possibilities for your family?*

PART FIVE

Beyond Our Back Door

Chapter Twenty-Two

Cornwall

Remember that sometimes not getting what you want
is a wonderful stroke of luck.
—Dalai Lama

There really is a place in the world called Land's End. It's not just a sportswear catalog. Land's End is the westernmost tip of England, located in the county of Cornwall, and was at one time the end of the known world for inhabitants of Britain. Going beyond our back door with a child with chronic illness sometimes feels like we are leaving the known world. We expose ourselves to more risk when we step out of the familiar into the unknown. We learn and grow in immeasurable ways when we encounter challenges that push us to continue stepping into hope.

We weren't planning on going to Cornwall that spring of Austin's fifth-grade year. The fifth graders at the American School of London traveled to Calshot, a coastal village in southern England, for their annual week away. Like their fourth-grade trip, this weeklong adventure emphasized relationship building and experiencing time away from home. This trip placed an additional focus on the biodiversity of the seashore.

My son's fourth-grade teacher stops me in the hall. We became friendly during the year he taught Austin, and especially after the four-day Outward Bound-style camp trip, which I attended as a chaperone.

"I'm hearing rumors you won't be allowed to chaperone the fifth-grade trip after all."

My jaw drops and my eyes open wide as I try to process what I've just heard. I have accompanied my son on every school field trip—both in the US and in the UK—since his T1D diagnosis. I'm stunned.

"You know no parents ever attend that trip," he says, breaking the silence. "I spoke up on your behalf last year, and again this week, informing the teachers and administrators that T1D is more complex than they can handle without you."

"Are they sending a nurse?" I venture, knowing nurses aren't usually sent on this trip either.

"I don't think so," my friend replies. "It doesn't look good. You need to speak with Austin's teacher, and also the principal."

I thank him and make my way through the school, collecting my children to walk home. The trip is in less than a month. I don't understand why intelligent people can so stubbornly hold onto their fixed ideas about my child's health needs as though they were the experts. They don't understand the complexity of the disease, nor do they understand the risks.

The day of our scheduled meeting arrives. I insisted my husband leave work to join us. As much as I hate to admit it, I fear being taken advantage of by the two men who think they understand our son's needs better than my husband and I do. Two on two, I reason, Jon and I present a stronger defense.

The air is thick as we state our case calmly and logically to the principal and the fifth-grade teacher. "Who will do the nighttime blood tests? Who will change his site for his insulin pump? What will you do if his blood sugar won't come down and he develops diabetic ketoacidosis, a life-threatening condition?"

I continue to pummel them with questions. The principal continues to resist me as he repeats there will be no parental chaperones on the trip.

I adjust my tack slightly.

"An adult must be trained to care for our son. Will you reconsider and send a nurse on the trip?"

"No, Mrs. O'Neil, we won't," he replies coolly. "That's not how we do things here."

"I don't understand why the school is willing to assume so much unnecessary risk. I've tried explaining the risks, but it doesn't seem to matter to you." My heart beats faster as I speak the ultimatum Jon and I had decided was to be our final option. "If you don't change your policy to something we can get comfortable with, then we won't be sending Austin on the trip."

The principal saves his strongest bullet for last. "The other family with a child with T1D has no problem sending their son. I don't understand why you're making such a big deal about it."

My blood is boiling now. As our son's parents, we are responsible for his care. We decide what feels safe and prudent for our son. In my gut I know this isn't safe.

"I'm sorry. You've left us no choice," I reply, standing up. "Austin won't be joining his classmates on the field trip this year."

You know your child better than anyone else does. You know her better than any doctor does. Better than any teacher does. And better than any school administrator ever will. You understand the complexity and risk inherent with your child's illness. You are your child's number one advocate, today and always.

You are your child's number one advocate,
today and always.

When we advocate for our children, we demonstrate to them that we are their champions. When we fight for their rights, we teach them never to give up without trying. Knowing we have their back, our children can rest in the hope for their future.

Sometimes we have to raise our voices as advocates even before we fully understand the complexities of our child's disease. Barely two months into Austin's diabetes, I had to work with his new school to develop the first of thirteen annual 504 Plans. Every year, with the return to school, you too will need to develop your own 504 Plan that clearly identifies concessions granted to your child to create a safe and learning-appropriate environment. Your plan may include provision for access to medicine, food, nursing care or an aide, as well as accommodations for test taking or missed work. Every child is different, and every 504 Plan is different.

Advocating doesn't end at the schoolyard. You may need to educate and advocate at dance class, youth sports teams, your house of worship, or summer camp to ensure your child is not discriminated against because of her health constraints. As your child grows, you will continue advocating for him as you apply for accommodations for standardized testing and perhaps accommodations for housing or academic support while at college. It's our responsibility to understand the real risks, as distinct from our own fears, and be able to present them clearly when asking for concessions for our children.

When we fight for our children's rights, it can be a struggle to find the balance between being assertive and overbearing. If we're pushed against a wall, like I was before the fifth-grade field trip, it's tempting to push back, loudly and defensively. I've never found pushing back defensively to be effective. I look instead to temper boldness and courage with grace and respect. Sometimes it's boldness I lack. Other times I could do with a larger helping of grace and respect in my communication style.

We model for our children how to navigate conflict. Soon my son will be his own advocate. If the only example I give him is yelling and screaming to get what I want, then he will either pattern himself after me or he might not be inclined to self-advocate at all. On the other hand, if he never sees me act with enough boldness to push back respectfully, he may learn he has to accept every limitation placed upon him. The way I advocate for my child today teaches him how to self-advocate in the future.

When our plans fail, it's tempting to get stuck in the mire, venting our complaints to family and friends, decrying the ones who block our way forward. We may also speak too openly about the dangers and limitations in our children's lives, making them feel scared, weak, or vulnerable. I don't want my child to feel defined by his illness. When we choose our words carefully, we can encourage our children, even when our plans fail. Perhaps in those times, more than any other, our words have the power to transport our children to a place of hope.

Like many aspects of raising a child with chronic illness, advocating for their needs provides us ample opportunity to practice letting go of expectations. Despite our best efforts and the logic of our arguments, the outcome of our advocacy is never guaranteed. I wish I could say I no longer struggle with disappointment over unmet expectations. But I do. In my meeting with the middle school principal and teacher, it took great self-control not to hurl insults at them when they denied our request. Instead of thinking about myself, I thought about Austin. I don't want teachers and administrators to transfer their annoyance with me to their treatment of him. Showing my disappointment while remaining respectful is in the long-term best interest of my child.

I want my child to know he is my number one
priority; winning a fight is not.

I want my child to know *he* is my number one priority; winning a fight is not.

We don't always get our way, but we can always hold out hope for another way. When Plan A fails, we need to get creative and pivot to Plan B.

I had only a few weeks to devise our Plan B. I was not about to let Austin miss an opportunity to explore the English seaside just because of his illness. We would make our own field trip, I reasoned. Alexander had a high school baseball tournament that weekend, so he stayed in London with a friend while the rest of us traveled together to Cornwall. We explored St. Michael's Mount—a rocky island whose only access road magically appears and disappears with the changing tides. Austin and Alicia delighted in the town of Penzance, the mythical home of the pirates in Gilbert and Sullivan's comic opera *The Pirates of Penzance*. We bought them two foam swords and watched them play at pirates the rest of the day. Finally, we arrived at Land's End, the supposed end of the known world.

At the end of the weekend, Jon and Alicia traveled back to London while Austin and I continued on to the wilder northern coast of Cornwall. The cliffs cascaded down to the sea as if someone had sliced the land away from some other rocky outcrop, setting the island called Britain adrift in the sea. Verdant green grass waved along the tops of the cliffs as wildflowers dressed in sunny yellow, pale pink, and lacey white decorated the hillsides. The Cornwall coast took our breath away with its rugged beauty. Our refrain quickly became, "Who needs Calshot when you can have Cornwall?"

We stayed there for three days, filling our daylight hours with bike rides along the tops of the cliffs and playing in the sand on the beach below. Austin brought a little pack of soldiers with him and spent hours reenacting the D-Day Battle of Normandy, the jagged cliffs having reminded him of the Norman landscape. We played tennis and he even enjoyed a few rounds of bungee jumping over a trampoline. In the evenings we lingered over delicious dinners at the hotel before making our way to the lounge to play backgammon, a game I taught him during those quiet evenings by the sea. He brought his guitar along, so some evenings he serenaded me before settling into a bedtime movie together.

We accomplished the trip's stated goals—relationship building, time away from home, and the study of seaside biodiversity.

When we returned to London, we learned that while we were happily tucked into our beach hotel in Cornwall, the other student with T1D had been hospitalized with diabetic ketoacidosis the first night of the school trip. As caregivers we always need to trust our gut and advocate boldly for our child's well-being.

When we arrived at Land's End, I noticed the mile marker sign pointing across the sea. It read, *New York: 3047 miles*. Land's End is not in fact the end of the world. It simply points to another land with other possibilities. A fitting reminder that even when we think we've reached the end and can do no more, love never declares defeat. Love always finds another way.

Heart to Heart

- *In what ways do you demonstrate to your child that you are his advocate?*

- *How do you respond when your advocacy efforts fail?*

- *How can you demonstrate to your child that there's always another way through a problem? How might your words and actions convey that even a blocked road is not the end of the world?*

Chapter Twenty-Three

France

*You cannot get through a single day without having an impact
on the world around you. What you do makes a difference,
and you have to decide what kind of difference you want to make.*
—Dr. Jane Goodall

If a picture paints a thousand words, then the photo I hold in my hand tells the story of these next one thousand words. Nestled in my photo album between other pictures taken at the Chateau St. Germain de Livet in Normandy, France, this photo draws my eyes to linger on it a little longer than on the others. It's one of many photos Alexander snapped that day. I slip it out of its little plastic sleeve to get a clearer look. Sunglasses shield my eyes from the mid-July sun that glistens on my hair and illuminates the garden scene beyond. One hand holds my cell phone to my ear while I use the other to animate my speech. Captured in profile, I exude an air of calm and peace. While the image may feign calm, there was nothing peaceful about those moments.

I close my eyes, and the entire one-thousand-word story comes rushing back to me.

We're on one of our occasional trips to France, visiting the next generation of the family I had lived with when I was a college student in Paris. We two families had our first sons a few months apart when Jon and I were living in France ten years later, and all six of our children line up perfectly in age.

It's a warm, clear Thursday morning as Valerie and I return from visiting an art exhibition in a neighboring town. With six children between us, the only real way to have a few moments of quiet is to leave the house and put the dads in charge. The unexpected ring of my phone interrupts our pleasant conversation. Austin's thirteen-year-old voice breaks in after my tentative, "Hello?"

"My pump broke." In the background I hear the sound of his pump alarm signaling there's a major malfunction. "It broke while we were playing in the yard."

Visions of adolescent children tackling each other over possession of a soccer ball float across my mind. "Did you fall on it?" I ask.

"I don't know. It just broke," was all he cared to say.

"We'll be right home," I assure him. "I'll try to get it to work."

My efforts at troubleshooting Austin's pump fail. We can't even get the alarm to stop sounding unless we remove the batteries. The vacation bliss of a few hours before evaporates as I step into emergency management mode. First, a shot of the long-acting insulin he used before going on a pump. Next, changing out his daily supply bag to contain syringes and insulin rather than extra pump supplies. Finally, I begin the calls to try to locate a replacement pump. I'm grateful we thought to set up our phones for international calling on this trip.

This is the only time we ever traveled a long distance without a spare pump. Pump manufacturers typically allow families to borrow a loaner pump when traveling on vacation for emergencies just like this. My son's pump manufacturer was exiting the diabetes business, so they no longer had a supply of loaner pumps. Thankfully, his pump is still under warranty, so they have to provide us with a pump to replace the broken one. But could they get it to us by tomorrow? We leave at daybreak on Saturday for the long drive to a remote village in Provence, in the south of France.

Calls ring out to the UK, Germany, and France as they try to locate a spare pump for us. The waiting between the myriad phone calls is the hardest part. If I can keep someone on the phone, I convince myself, I can persuade him to loan us a pump. I continue making calls even as we explore the region as tourists. Alexander snaps a photo of me, phone to my ear, capturing the memory of an unresolved crisis. Finally, thirty hours after our drama began to unfold, they locate a pump in Paris that we can borrow for the rest of our trip. Relieved, I call our leasing agent for the house in Provence, and she agrees to receive the pump at her home address. With no weekend deliveries in her town, we'll have the pump on Monday, four days after our saga began.

Living beyond the borders of our back door requires enormous flexibility and creativity. Life outside routine invites unpredictability. Even the most thoughtful planning can't prepare us for every possible risk. And even when nothing goes terribly wrong, we caregivers never get a vacation from our child's illness.

Living beyond the borders of our back door requires enormous flexibility and creativity. Life outside routine invites unpredictability.

That was one of the hardest things for me to accept—that I never got a vacation from T1D. I know I shouldn't complain; I'm not the one living with the disease after all. But as my son's caregiver, the weight of worry and the need to always be alert were burdens I longed to lay down, even if only for a short time. I grew so weary of the frequent interruptions and resented never getting a vacation from T1D.

I've had to troubleshoot frequently as my son's caregiver, especially when on vacation. But this time—finding an insulin pump in a foreign country—felt like finding a needle in a haystack. I needed rest, but rest is often elusive for caregivers.

The tedium of constant troubleshooting weighs heavy. Round and round the caregiver's wheel we go again. Interruptions. Troubleshooting. Decision making. Taking action. Waiting. Observing. Worrying. Fearing. Releasing control. The caregiver's wheel never stops. Repetition is in the DNA of caregiving.

Even on vacation I remain the caregiver, the troubleshooter. Vacation means late dinners and restaurant meals laden with hidden fats and carbohydrates. I sleep less and test blood sugars more on vacation than when we stay at home. These nights, when I realize I'm the only one in my family who appears stressed, my heart brims with anger and jealousy.

Frustration rings out in the dissonance between our expectation of what we want and the reality of what is.

Frustration rings out in the dissonance between our expectation of what we want and the reality of what is.

Why can't I relax like my husband and kids? Is there a way to balance vigilant caregiving with a less worry-filled mindset? We need to be vigilant in caring for our children with chronic illness. It's an awesome responsibility we carry. But how do we find pockets of rest amidst the stress of being a caregiver?

Accepting the unpredictability of our child's illness is a good place to start. We need realistic expectations so we don't condemn ourselves whenever we fail to control every element of our child's disease. It's unhealthy to feel like a failure because things don't go as we've planned. Expecting interruptions allows us to mentally prepare for them so they don't completely unhinge us. Of course, to expect interruptions means we have to let go of perfectionism, at least while we're on vacation. I wish I had practiced this when my son was younger; it might have helped me relax a little more. Holding our expectations more loosely helps us handle the uncertainties and unexpected surprises of chronic illness with less fear and greater grace. The more I offer myself grace, the more I project hope to my child.

In all my concern to keep my son safe and healthy, I think I sometimes forgot how to laugh. We can be so focused on not letting down our guard and not neglecting our responsibility as our child's caregiver that we invite fear to eclipse joy. Caregiving is serious business, but when we lead with anxiety, we teach our children to worry. We do well to create moments of levity even in the hard times. As the saying goes, *laughter is the best medicine*. Laughing increases blood flow, improves the function of blood vessels, and relaxes the body. Laughter actually does relieve stress and tension. Learning to laugh together in our trials teaches our families patience, love, and flexibility, and helps us reduce stress in the process.

One of the best gifts we can give our kids is demonstrating our confidence that, with a little ingenuity, we can sort things out. Even if they don't vocalize their concerns, chances are they too worry during a crisis. Not having his pump weighed heavy on Austin's mind. He didn't like being back on shots and was anxious to return to his preferred form of insulin therapy. In the four days spent waiting for his new pump, Austin asked me repeatedly if it had arrived. When life takes a surprising turn, modeling calm amidst the storm fans the embers of hope for our children.

I want my family to live a full life. I don't want our life to become too small because I'm afraid of stepping out of my routine. Welcoming risk means accepting the unpredictability of caregiving in new environments. I shield hope for my child when I embrace life despite the risks.

Remembering the blessings in my life and choosing gratitude over worry helps me reframe situations that don't go according to plan. I can look at that photo of me in the garden at the chateau in France and remember a story of crisis, fear, uncertainty, caregiver fatigue, frustration, and vacation interruption. Or I can replace my tired eyes with eyes of gratitude and remember a very different story. I can remember the story of quick thinking, caring friends, helpful strangers, and a crisis averted.

We finally receive the pump on Monday afternoon, after a full day of sightseeing. I remove the pump from its box, press the *on* button, and wait for it to light up. I laugh and shake my head in disbelief as I discover all the words on the pump screen are *in French!* I chuckle that it never crossed my mind I would be programming the pump in French. I'm extremely grateful we weren't sent a pump from Germany!

Before preparing dinner, I sit at the long kitchen table and program *la pompe à insuline* in French. Austin is relieved to be wearing his pump again and rather amused by the funny words on the screen. He knows his pump so intimately that he can maneuver the prompts and screens without needing to read the words. Just to be cautious, though, he has me look over his shoulder as he moves through the inputs.

Thankful hearts are fertile ground for hope to flourish.

We take a moment as a family to soak in our thankfulness for how this story ended. We experienced the kindness of strangers who went out of their way to help our son. We recognize the miracle of locating a spare insulin pump on short notice and receiving it in a remote corner of France. We marvel that the pump is programmed in the only other language I know how to read and speak. Thankful hearts are fertile ground for hope to flourish.

Heart to Heart

- *How do you respond to unexpected problems and interruptions stemming from your child's illness?*

- *How do you experience rest from the burden of full-time caregiving? How could you modify your expectations to have more restful vacations?*

- *What steps might you take to balance your vigilance as a caregiver with an intention to worry less?*

Chapter Twenty-Four

Costa Rica

In spite of…all our miseries, which touch us, which grip us by the throat,
we have an instinct which we cannot repress and which lifts us up.
—Blaise Pascal

Our family has enjoyed many relaxing vacations post-diagnosis that presented us with no unexpected challenges. Our trip to Costa Rica when Austin was sixteen years old was not one of those vacations. Some stories are almost as painful in the retelling as they were in the experience itself. This is one of those stories.

I had compared our school calendars the prior fall and discovered with delight that all three children shared the same spring break. With children in two different high schools in Pennsylvania and one in college in North Carolina, this seemed like a minor miracle. We leapt at the chance to get away together like we used to when the kids were younger. The children wanted warm weather; Jon and I wanted a novel location. A week in Costa Rica exploring the beaches and rainforest jungles sounded like the perfect spot for exotic exploration and relaxation.

We arrive at our seaside hotel late in the afternoon, wasting no time to take our first plunge in the cool waters of its spacious pool. The following day we wander down the beach about a mile away for a late

179

lunch at a beachside restaurant nestled into a grove of swaying palm trees. It's a picture-perfect oasis sheltering us from the heat of the Pacific coast.

The boys eat quickly and ask to be excused to go swimming while the rest of us finish eating. A few minutes later Austin returns to the table, complaining of feeling shaky. A quick blood test reveals his blood sugar is dangerously low at thirty-seven. He had just given himself twelve units of insulin for his lunch, so I know his blood sugar will continue to drop if he doesn't get some sugar quickly. After drinking an entire sixteen-ounce bottle of Coke, his blood sugar rises only to sixty. *Why won't his blood sugar go up?* I wonder, concern mounting. A few minutes later Austin's nausea sets in and I have my answer. Austin has food poisoning.

Our idyllic setting quickly turns into a living nightmare. Because of the food poisoning, Austin's body will never use the twelve units of insulin to metabolize the carbohydrates in his lunch; the insulin will only work to drive his blood sugar lower and lower. Once the vomiting sets in, his blood sugar will continue to plummet. Coke and juice are no longer viable options for us to elevate his blood sugar—they will only make him vomit more.

I need his glucagon—the emergency shot contained in the long, slim red box. Glucagon elevates blood sugar when someone with T1D can't eat or drink. I have dutifully filled his glucagon prescription for the past eleven years, leaving one at home, another at school, and taking one with us on every vacation, but I've never had to use one before. I took it to Costa Rica with us, but I didn't put it in our beach bag. It's back at the hotel.

Hastily we formulate a plan. Jon and Alexander will run back to the hotel. Alexander will race back with the glucagon while Jon navigates the bumpy, windy roads back to the restaurant by car. They take off on a race against time, sprinting down the rocky coast in bare feet. Austin's projectile vomiting begins almost as soon as they leave us.

"Puedo ayudarle?" the waitress says to me. I understand not a word.

"I don't speak Spanish," I reply. "My son has diabetes—la diabete," I offer, wondering if this word comes anywhere close to the Spanish word for diabetes.

"Nécessita un médico?" The words continue to flow—theirs in Spanish, mine in English.

A small crowd begins to enfold us. The scene is pure chaos as the group of locals tries to offer assistance to the poor gringo mother and her vomiting son. The only real communication between us is my terror-filled face met with their glances of compassion. We all feel helpless.

The sun is setting low in the sky when Alexander finally returns, breathless and with gashes in his feet from the rocky coast. With trembling hands I open the red box and mix the powder and liquid together. In the dim light I inject my son with the life-saving medicine. The vomiting continues as another twenty minutes pass before Jon arrives with the car to take us back to the hotel. Austin's blood sugar increases slightly, but not enough to feel safe. I don't have another glucagon.

At the hotel we ask the concierge to call for a doctor. He arrives about an hour after we return to the hotel and hooks Austin up to an IV-drip of dextrose and saline to elevate his blood sugar and flush out his ketones. Austin continues vomiting throughout the night. He is in diabetic ketoacidosis. The doctor stays with us most of the night and returns the following day to discover Austin has developed a fever.

"Food poisoning can cause a fever, but we have to rule out appendicitis," the doctor tells us. "We need to get your son to the private hospital in San Jose immediately in case he needs surgery."

Terrified at the prospect of my son having an emergency appendectomy in a developing country, I hastily pack our bags while the doctor makes the necessary arrangements. With Jon, Alexander, and Alicia following in the rental car, the doctor, Austin, and I travel by ambulance the four hours down to the capital.

Fear locked eyes with me during those first twenty-four hours and wouldn't let go. I feared for my son's life as I never had before. Fear is the enemy of the soul. Seeing only fear, we reject all that is good and beautiful and sacred in the world. To lock eyes with fear, seeing nothing but brokenness ahead, is to reject hope.

Fear is the enemy of the soul. Seeing only fear, we reject all that is good and beautiful and sacred in the world.

During the journey to the hospital, as my son feared for his life and all I could envision were the risks involved in emergency surgery in Costa Rica, I wrestled once again with God. When Austin was first diagnosed with T1D, questions came hard and without reprieve. One resounded louder than the others: *How could a good God allow bad things to happen, especially to those who love him?* Finding no answer to my liking, I walked away from my faith, and for two years I wore my disappointment with God like a heavy blanket, wrapping it tighter and tighter around me like armor.

It took time to rebuild my faith on a firmer foundation—one where I no longer demanded God be a benevolent genie willing to grant me an endless supply of Three Wishes. I could only develop a new faith—a faith that's willing to accept the good from God as well as the bad—when I began to let go of my anger. Looking at life through angry eyes takes all the truth out of the world.

My spiritual crisis was different this time. I had learned enough about control to know I didn't have any. I had seen myself steeped in hidden anger for years and knew anger didn't solve anything. Love, I had discovered, was the only thing greater than fear, greater than anger, and more powerful than a loss of control. In that ambulance I experienced what can only be described as a spiritual epiphany. I released my insistence on controlling life and death, on controlling the disease, and—dare I say—on controlling God. I released Austin from my tight grasp to an unknown future. I had come full circle from my response when Austin was first diagnosed with T1D. At diagnosis I let go of God and clutched my son for dear life, and my world became dark and hopeless. In Costa Rica I let go of Austin and held onto God, and my heart flooded with peace.

I don't know what pain you carry deep within as a result of your child's illness. Perhaps it's an unresolved spiritual crisis like I experienced. Perhaps it's an inability to trust—yourself, your spouse, your child's future, or the world in general. Maybe you can't shake the fear—always simmering below the surface—that convinces you your family isn't *safe*. Perhaps you're still mourning the death of a dream. Whatever pain you still hold onto, would you be willing to take it into the light and examine it for what it is?

Austin didn't have appendicitis, but he spent the next three days in the hospital recuperating. During those days I had a lot of time to think not just about my emotional health as my son's caregiver, but also about the level of preparedness we need to take when traveling. I thought we were well prepared for this trip, but I discovered there was more I could do to keep my son safe while on vacation.

I've learned to make a contingency plan. It's critical to know where the nearest hospital is located and how to get there in an emergency. I now know to inquire of the hotel staff before arriving if there's a doctor who makes house calls. This is especially important when traveling in the developing world. I can't imagine how our trip might have turned out had the doctor not been there to treat my son at our hotel.

I now take double of *all* medical supplies, especially when traveling internationally or to remote places in the US. We can't assume we'll be able to buy what we need; some medical supplies are simply not available in other countries. I discovered at the hospital that there had been no glucagon in the entire country of Costa Rica for over ten years because the drug is too expensive. I also learned the hard way to always have our full emergency kit *readily available*. Taking it on vacation but leaving it in the hotel room does us no good in an emergency.

This was my son's first hospitalization. I discovered pretty quickly that I knew more about T1D than the attending physicians. They wanted to remove Austin's insulin pump and try to regulate his blood sugars using an outdated approach. By demonstrating my knowledge and confidence in managing Austin's T1D, and treating the hospital staff with respect, the doctors came to trust me enough to let me manage Austin's diabetes while they took care of the rest.

Crises are like school exams. They test what we've learned and how we're processing what we've experienced.

Crises are like school exams. They test what we've learned and how we're processing what we've experienced. In a crisis, we have to act fast. In those moments, we discover how much we've learned. After the crisis, in the quiet moments of reflection, we can take stock of our emotional health. On the beach, I had to act fast. My son's life was on the line. In the ambulance, with nothing more I could do, and nothing but an uncertain future ahead of us, I discovered all of life is a precious gift, even when it gets messy and hard. I came to terms with my son's mortality, and my own. And I finally accepted I was not in control of my life or my son's. Relinquishing the façade of control opened my heart to more freely love my son.

Heart to Heart

- *Reflect on a crisis you experienced with your child. How do you respond tactically in a crisis? How do you respond emotionally during and after a crisis?*

- *What emotions or fears have you buried that tend to rise to the surface during a crisis?*

- *How might you begin to hold those fears more loosely so they don't have such a stranglehold over you?*

Chapter Twenty-Five

College

You gain strength, courage, and confidence by every experience
in which you really stop to look fear in the face.
You must do the thing you think you cannot do.
—ELEANOR ROOSEVELT

"No, I don't want you to drive," I snap at my husband, my hands white-knuckling the wheel at ten and two. I can't just sit in this car, useless, for the next two-and-a-half hours. I need something to do. How did everything go so terribly wrong? This was not the college move-in I had envisioned.

Ask any parent of a child with T1D what day they most dread in their child's life, and they will tell you "the day I drop my child off at college." That's the day we cease being our child's fulltime caregiver and let go of any remaining vestige of control.

The tears flow freely now as anger and frustration melt into sorrow and resignation. I had prepared well. I had put every safety net in place. I found a CVS pharmacy—like Austin used at home—within walking distance from his dorm. I had arranged a medical power of attorney. I put the process in place for Austin to receive accommodations in case of diabetes-related issues interfering with his academic work. There was just this one niggling concern. He never heard from his roommate.

We arrived on campus the day before move-in to have dinner with all the families from our hometown. We have just enough time to drop off Austin's prescriptions at the CVS before joining our friends at the restaurant down the street for dinner. Approaching the storefront, we notice the cardboard on the windows before we see the sign—*Store Closed. Visit our new location at 350 N 10th Street.* How can this be? The store was open just a few weeks ago. The new pharmacy is too far for my son to go on foot.

My mind is still swirling as we settle into the restaurant, greeting our friends and congratulating one another on their child's exciting future. I'm glad we arrived a day ahead; I'll need time to find my son another pharmacy.

The students and their siblings sit at one long table while their proud parents sit at the only other table in the private dining space where we've gathered. I glance over at our children, thankful that as my son steps into life without me, he has a ready group of friends by his side. My blissful thoughts last but a moment. I look up from scanning the menu to discover Austin standing next to me.

He whispers in my ear, "My roommate withdrew. He's not coming."

I quickly turn toward him. "What do you mean? How do you know that?"

"One of the kids found the list of incoming freshmen posted online, and his name isn't on the list. I'm gonna be all alone."

The last thing my son or I wanted was for him to be alone. If blood sugars fall rapidly during sleep, an attentive roommate can literally be a lifesaver. I had carefully explained all of this to the Housing Office earlier this summer.

"We'll sort it out. Don't worry."

But I do worry. I toss and turn all night long, fearful of the consequences if I can't sort out these two unexpected problems. I have a lead on a new pharmacy, but I won't rest easy until we see it. The morning move-in goes well. I hope it's a harbinger of quickly finding a new roommate and a new pharmacy. My calls to the Housing Office have to wait until after we unpack Austin's things and leave his dorm room. As it turns out, Austin's dorm doesn't get cell service. A third safety net cut out from underneath us.

I call the Housing Office and plead Austin's case. They are resolute. There will be no rearranging of roommates at this late date unless another student requests a change in the next few weeks. My apprehension continues to rise.

Minutes after returning from the new pharmacy we discovered, an orientation counselor appears at Austin's door. With a broad smile, she declares it's time for the new students to follow her to Orientation. "Mom and Dad," she announces," it's time for you to go home." There was no five-minute warning. College came calling for my son, and I could hold onto him no longer.

Our goodbyes are hasty. Are there not a million final cautionary words I need to impart to my son? Can't I at least have a few moments of privacy without the watchful gaze of the orientation counselor to tell my son how much I love him? We share a quick hug and an *I love you* before he disappears down the hall amidst a sea of other happy freshmen.

Stunned, Jon and I look at each other as we process what just happened. In a fog, we find our car and begin to drive away from campus.

"Stop!" I shout from the passenger seat. "What are we doing? There's not a single person on Austin's side of campus who even knows he has T1D. All his friends from home are in the other dorms. He has no roommate. I didn't get to meet the RA yet. I didn't do everything I was supposed to do before leaving him. Turn back!"

We drive back to campus, making our way to the lawn outside Austin's dorm. It looks like a ghost town compared to a few hours ago. I stop one student in an official-looking orange T-shirt.

"Do you know who the RA is up on the second floor of Vedder Hall?" I ask, trying to choke back my tears. "I need to find my son's RA."

"No, I'm sorry, I don't," she replies. "But some of the freshmen are on the other side of the building for Orientation; you could look over there for your son's group."

We thank her as she dashes off. I envy her lightheartedness. Jon and I both know we won't walk around the building and risk being seen by Austin. He would be mortified to be singled out as the student with the lurking parents. He feels ready for his independence, even if I'm not quite ready to let him go. I ask Jon for the car keys. I need something other than my perceived failure as Austin's caregiver to occupy my mind during the drive home.

Perhaps you picked up this book and scanned the chapter titles, and before reading all the preceding chapters, you turned to this one in particular. You turned here because you too dread the day you will have to drop your child off at college, and you wanted some assurance everything would be okay. I'm sorry my story didn't go as well as either of us would have liked. I know it would be much easier for you to read a story that came off without a hitch. But life doesn't always turn out exactly like we want it to, does it?

Many of us yearn for a smooth road, one where our carefully orchestrated plans operate like clockwork. What if we re-envision the benefits of problems arising on our watch? When we face challenges—even major crises like the ones my family has experienced—our children have the opportunity to witness firsthand the manner in which we problem solve. At times I've been so focused on protecting my son from experiencing unforeseen problems related to his T1D that I've forgotten how much we can all learn when faced with setbacks. Solving problems with our children teaches them how to face a crisis with courage and resilience, pushing through it until they find a solution.

Next to me at dinner the night before move-in sat the dean of the School of Management. Our friends who had organized the evening were both alums of the university, so they had invited him to join us to welcome the students and families. The dean's presence at the table was a gift of pure grace to my family. He told me of a new, family-owned pharmacy opening just that week within walking distance of campus. The following day we met the pharmacist-owner, who assured us he would take good care of Austin. Not only would they deliver Austin's medicines to his dorm, but also, as we were leaving, the pharmacist gave us his cell phone number in case we ever needed to reach him. Failing at my plan to find the "perfect pharmacy" was actually a blessing in disguise.

When I moved my son into college, I once again fell prey to an if-then mentality—if I do everything right to prepare my child for college, then nothing will go wrong and he will be safe. We can make the best plans in the world, but they don't guarantee our children will be safe. Likewise, just because things don't go according to plan doesn't mean we've failed as our child's caregiver. There's potentially more value in what we demonstrate to our children when things go wrong than when everything goes right.

> *There's potentially more value in what we demonstrate to our children when things go wrong than when everything goes right.*

We long for college move-in day to unfold seamlessly, for that allows us to remain under the illusion that we're still in control. Yet one of our primary roles as our child's parent is to prepare him for independence. For us, this also means working ourselves out of the job as our child's primary caregiver. The tension between teaching our child independence and desiring perfection in his care pulls at us constantly. To let them grow in independence requires us to accept greater "user error." Letting go also requires us to accept that our child might not do things the same way we do. Accepting their way of managing their disease after years of being in charge can be difficult. But if we've built a solid relationship with our children when they're young, they may just rehire us as their consultants when they're adults.

Training ourselves to let go is harder than teaching them to be independent. They are undoubtedly more ready to fly solo than we are prepared to let them go. We do have to prepare as best as possible for our child's departure to college, but the most important part of the preparations happens slowly, over the course of many years together. We teach them what we know about their disease and how to manage it. We teach them what to do in a crisis by modeling for them our own resourcefulness. When unwelcomed surprises interrupt our plans, we shelter hope for them.

There comes a time when we have to trust our child is ready, even if we don't feel ready to let them test their wings.

There comes a time when we have to trust our child is ready, even if we don't feel ready to let them test their wings. Even if the goodbye isn't what we had envisioned. Even if we still have items left on our college prep to-do list. We need to remember we've been teaching and training our child all along. They have been watching and learning, waiting for the moment for us to step aside so they can take flight.

Heart to Heart

- *How have you experienced fear of letting go of your child as he goes off on his own?*

- *What have you learned from the setbacks you have experienced in your carefully orchestrated plans regarding your child's well-being?*

- *In what ways might you shelter hope for your child when obstacles threaten to derail your plans?*

Chapter Twenty-Six

911

All shall be well, and all shall be well,
and all manner of thing shall be well.
—JULIAN OF NORWICH

I open my eyes and fumble on the bedside table in my dimly lit bedroom for my phone. The time reads 6:48 a.m. Time to get my groggy self out of bed. I notice two texts from Austin came at 1:58 a.m. He's a freshman at college; my heart begins to beat faster. I press my index finger on his name to open the texts.

"Just threw up." "I have a stomach virus."

Instantly I'm awake and on diabetes-mom overdrive. Stomach viruses require careful monitoring because of the risk of free-falling blood sugars and the development of a large volume of ketones. My son has never experienced a stomach virus or diabetic ketoacidosis without my support. Fear courses through my body.

I try calling him, hoping he will miraculously have cell service in his dorm room. His is the only dorm on campus where Verizon users have no cell service. We rely on FaceTime or texting to communicate with one another this year. I send him multiple texts that disappear into the cell waves. For an agonizingly long and frightful twenty-five minutes, my attempts to reach my son remain unanswered. *He must have fallen asleep,* I conclude.

He has no roommate I can text. The Housing Office was never able to find him a replacement for his roommate who withdrew just before the start of the year. I scratch out a text to the RA, who has already proven to be of little help in matters relating to T1D. I don't hold out much hope of him awakening Austin.

My mind slips into a dangerous place of dark imaginings. I picture my long, lean son, all six-foot-four of him, curled up in bed. He drifts off to sleep, having forgotten to check for ketones. Perhaps with the dehydration so common in vomiting, he didn't even have enough urine to pee on a strip to test for ketones. Has he remembered to test his blood sugars throughout these five hours? Was his blood sugar high enough to safely fall off to sleep?

The questions assault my mind as I picture my son sleeping off the final bout of vomiting, his crop of blond hair gently caressing his pillow. What will happen to him if he falls asleep with large ketones? Will he ever wake up?

My phone lights up at 7:15 a.m. It's Austin.

"Austin!" I cry, still not sure what I will find on the other end of the phone. "Are you alright?"

"Yeah. I'm okay."

I exhale the breath I realize I've been holding for close to thirty minutes. "Where are you?" are the only words I can think to string together.

"I'm outside Vedder. I'm waiting for the ambulance to take me to the hospital. I called 911 as soon as I got outside."

"Did you get my texts? I was so worried you had fallen asleep, and I didn't know how to reach you," I add with a catch in my throat.

"Yeah, sorry. I was throwing up for five hours and had large ketones. I knew I had to get to the hospital, so I took a quick shower." He pauses before adding with a slight chuckle, "I was using trash bags to throw up in, and one of them leaked. I needed to get cleaned up."

I imagine my son, weak from his virus and the vomiting, waiting outside with a wet head in an early morning February chill, calling 911. My heart breaks as I long to hold him tight.

"I'm so proud of you, Austin. You did exactly the right things—you tested for ketones and you knew when you needed to call for help." I remain on the phone with him until the ambulance arrives.

"The ambulance is here, Mom. Gotta go."

"Okay," I reply. "Text me when you get there. I'll get changed and be on my way. I'll see you in the ER in just under three hours."

I breathe deeply, inhaling relief, exhaling thanksgiving. My son is okay. He's more than okay; he handled his first solo flight like a seasoned veteran.

Emergencies are by definition unexpected, dangerous, and require our immediate attention. Because they are unpredictable, advance preparedness is essential. Like a skilled soldier trained from years of repetition by a competent leader, our children learn how to respond in an emergency as they develop the behaviors we drill into them.

During my son's high school years, I developed a few pat phrases that I used over and over again. I wanted him to be so familiar with these instructions that he could hear my voice in his head when he was in college. The phrase I used most frequently was "you throw up, you go to the hospital!" I made it clear he was not to handle bouts of vomiting on his own. There's too much at stake. Managing diabetes is difficult enough on the best of days. When sick, it can take more mental energy than a young adult can muster alone. I was never really sure he was listening though. I was relieved to discover he was!

When our children leave home for college, they may feel awkward about relying on us for help in the management of their illness. They may feel they have to manage everything independently. While we want to let them set the pace for how much they do on their own, we also want to assure them we're here for them when they get sick. Encouraging your child to communicate with you at the first sign of illness allows you to be another "set of eyes" from afar. Keeping a parent in the loop doesn't diminish your child's independence; it simply gives him an additional safety net.

Once they leave for college, we can no longer be with our children every day, so it's important they have a couple of friends who really have their back. These friends should have easy access to your child. Perhaps it's a roommate or a hall mate. Whoever your child selects must be bold enough to pound on her door and walk right in to check on her, especially if your child is sick. Be sure you have the names and phone numbers of your child's friends and they have yours. Having the RA's name and phone number isn't sufficient. Remember, RAs are employees of the school, so they will undoubtedly refer you to Campus Safety if you're concerned about your child's health.

Our children also need to know not to hesitate to call 911 when they realize they need help. The cost of an ambulance is well worth the peace of mind we have knowing our child is in capable hands.

One of the most important things I did before Austin left for college was to get a medical power of attorney for him. Because of HIPPA rules, having a medical POA on file is the only way medical personnel are legally allowed to speak to you about your adult child. When we dropped Austin at college that first fall, we took the medical POA to the university Health Office. They scanned it into their system and then *sent it electronically to the local hospital.* Because the medical POA was already at the local hospital, I was able to speak to the attending physician about Austin's care *from my car.*

We parents are so familiar with managing the nuances of our child's disease; we might not realize we have more current knowledge about the disease than the team of generalists in an ER. Because I had a medical POA for my son, I was able to guide the ER staff through the latest treatment protocol for diabetic ketoacidosis management. I explained the approach that the Children's Hospital of Philadelphia was using and begged them to try it. After consulting with an endocrinologist at the hospital, the attending physician called me back, thanked me, and said they would try the new protocol. This new approach hastened Austin's recovery by several hours.

Many children with chronic illness need to get an annual flu shot. Colleges and universities often hold flu clinics to administer these shots, and they often send email notifications to parents ahead of time. Remind your child to get the flu shot then, or to get one at home during fall break or Thanksgiving break.

Raising a child with T1D, my second most frequently used phrase was "always check for ketones when you're sick." We're taught to check for ketones when the blood sugar is too high, but people with T1D can get ketones even with a low or normal blood sugar. It was crucial that Austin knew to check for ketones. Ultimately, it was his large ketones—not the vomiting or a high blood sugar—that drove him to call 911. Your pat phrases may be different from mine, but developing a few simple, repeatable instructions may be the best tool you can give your child as he leaves home.

My son's dorm room resembles any other student's room—it's small, messy, and a little bit smelly—but if you look closely enough, you'll discover he has also readied his room for an emergency. His ketone strips are easily accessible in the large box of T1D supplies he totes with him to college each year. Somehow he always manages to squeeze this cumbersome box into a room already filled with standard-issue wooden beds, dressers, wardrobes, desks, and chairs. The trained eye will spot the six-inch-long red box—his emergency glucagon—like the one we had to use in Costa Rica. He always keeps it handy on the desk next to his bed where anyone could easily find it in an emergency. Also within reach are a couple of cans of Coke and Diet Coke. They're not for everyday consumption; they're also for emergency use only—for sipping to stay hydrated when vomiting.

We prepare our children by teaching them while they still live with us. Then we rest in the confidence that we've taught them to stand securely on their own two feet.

A little preparedness really does go a long way. We prepare our children by teaching them while they still live with us. Then we rest in the confidence that we've taught them to stand securely on their own two feet.

The day that began so stressfully for my son and me ended rather peacefully. My sister, Barb, lives fifteen minutes from the college. She and her husband met us at the hospital and welcomed us into their home that night. They nourished us with homemade chicken noodle soup and cocooned us in the warmth of their home and the embrace of their love. I slept like a baby, knowing my son would be okay. Hope had held steadfast and true.

Heart to Heart

- *How do you feel about your child leaving home one day?*

- *What key phrases or actions do you hope your child carries with him when he leaves home?*

- *How are you preparing your child for her eventual first crisis apart from you?*

Postlude

Hope Restored

My friends, love is better than anger. Hope is better than fear.
Optimism is better than despair. So let us be loving,
hopeful and optimistic. And we'll change the world.
—Jack Layton

I sit on a stone bench overlooking the Hudson River, waiting for my daughter. The shade cast by the lane of stately locust trees shades my face from the mid-August sun and keeps the stone remarkably cool. The seagulls stand sentry on a nearby pier, awaiting the arrival of passengers disembarking from Lower Manhattan. Their familiar shrill caw evokes images of the seaside in my mind, and I remember this harbor is not the gulls' permanent home. The waters of the Hudson don't terminate in the New York harbor; they spill into an expansive sea. The gulls do not belong in this hemmed-in space; they're just passing through. They belong in the vast openness of the seaside.

The river teems with activity. Vessels ferry people from one side of the river to the other, their horns resounding their deep-pitched blasts. Yachts travel down the river and into the harbor. Pleasure boats speed past as sailboats drift in their wake, catching the same breeze that gently blows the hair from my face.

I cast my gaze deeper into the harbor, and there I see her—Lady Liberty. I could circle the globe and not find a truer icon of hope. Sitting in the shadow of the Statue of Liberty, my thoughts turn to my mother, whose first glimpse of America was under the Great Lady's raised torch. For her immigrant family, and millions of others like them, their future was uncertain. But they were awash in hope.

Like all humanity, the future for us as caregivers is uncertain. But it is not without hope. The first dark days where hope appears cut off from our reach eventually open up, like the mouth of a river, into a life of abundant possibilities. Like those gulls, we aren't meant to remain locked in the harbor of despair. We too are just passing through this dark valley. Our futures are as uncertain as those of our Ellis Island forebears. But our hope is rock solid.

Why do we hope? We hope because we must. To deny hope is to remain clothed in a shroud of despair.

Sooner or later every one of us who bears human flesh will come face to face with suffering and despair. Our child's diagnosis with chronic illness has simply hastened our awareness of this reality. How we handle suffering and despair is largely influenced by our vision of hope.

Before our child's diagnosis we lived in the light of peace, joy, and expectation for our future. In the early days post-diagnosis, darkness threatened to block the light forever. Even a transcendent hope, buoyed by faith, can be damaged in these days. In time, we come to realize hope dwells in the shadow land. The deeper the shadow, the greater our need to trust in hope. You may not yet sense hope's presence—not much is visible in the darkest recesses of despair—but you can trust hope is waiting for you there. These passing shadows won't block the light forever. Living in hope is living in the confidence that the light will re-emerge to replace the darkness.

*In time, we come to realize hope dwells
in the shadow land. The deeper the shadow,
the greater our need to trust in hope.*

Hope draws us into its aura, beckoning us not to remain cloistered in the shadows. But hope doesn't come cheap. It costs us everything. Its wages are self-denial, release of control, acceptance of our new reality, forgiveness, courage, grace, and above all, love. If we are willing to do the hard work of loving this special family that has been entrusted to us, we may just see hope restored in ways we never imagined from where we stand today. Oh, it may look a little war-weary and tattered around the edges. Restored hope never looks exactly like our original vision of life.

Our new hope is not the stuff of schoolgirl dreams. This is not the longing for a new puppy on Christmas morn or yearning for the attentions of the cutest boy in class. Our new hope is firmly grounded in reality. Our hope is birthed out of the strength of will that accepts what is rather than demanding what will never be. To live in hope we must change the way we see and respond to the disappointments that threaten to consume us. To live in hope is to accept the fragility of life and choose to see its many benefits rather than its deficits.

Hope is not the guarantee that everything will work out as we had planned. In fact, it's just the opposite. To live in hope is to hold the circumstances of our lives loosely in our outstretched hands, without demanding life conform to our carefully ordered view of things. Hope is the steadied assurance that no matter how things turn out, we will be okay.

We can't live without hope. Hope is the air we breathe. We can choose to be held in hope's embrace rather than be shackled by despair. We can once again feel the expansiveness of hope coursing through our mind, body, and spirit. It's never too late to reach out in hope and begin again. I pray this vision of a hope-filled life encourages you to raise your child with grace, courage, and love, and that in the journey you too discover a heart beating with chronic hope.

Acknowledgments

The seeds for *Chronic Hope* were first sown while sitting across the table from my friend Christie Purifoy in a cozy garden shop café in southeastern Pennsylvania. She casually asked me a question writers often ask: "What do you want to write about next?" I had no fixed project in mind, so our conversation meandered to other topics. Toward the end of our time together, I offhandedly mentioned a recent speaking engagement where I shared with parents how to navigate the emotional stress of raising a child with chronic illness. Christie set down her nearly drained mug of tea, looked me in the eye, and pronounced the benediction.

"Write about that," she offered, and I knew I was sitting on holy ground. Thank you, Christie, for your attunement to the Spirit, for your encouragement of this book and of me as a writer, and mostly for your friendship.

Thank you, Ann Kroeker, for your early work with me in shaping the voice and structure of this book. Your gifts as a writing coach are exceptional!

Thanks to the friends and family who read early versions of my manuscript—Heather Giacoio, Carole Wells, Peggy Kepple, Donna Duffey, Renetta Reeves, Alicia O'Neil, and Jon O'Neil. I'm so grateful for your advice and encouragement.

Thank you, JDRF, for always supporting me on the journey of raising a child with T1D. Thank you for giving me the opportunity to share this story of hope through the TON Summits.

Thank you, Beyond Type 1, for so generously publishing my stories, many of which I have revised to become chapters within this book.

My deep thanks to David Hancock for your strong support of this book. To everyone at Morgan James Publishing and especially to my editor, Angie Kiesling, thank you for your diligent work throughout the publication process.

Thank you, Gary Scheiner, for your generosity in writing the Foreword for this book. Your compassion and expertise as you care for those impacted by T1D are a gift to the entire T1D community.

To my sisters, Barbara Gonsar and Betsy Shrader, thank you for living the early pages of this story with me and for your continued presence in my life.

To my husband, Jon, thank you for your unwavering belief in me and for your faithful encouragement of this project. To my children, Alexander, Austin, and Alicia, what a joy it is to be your mom. Thank you for cheering me on as I wrote this book. I love you up to the stars and back!

And my deepest thanks I offer to God. You are my rock, my light in the darkness, my true source of hope.

About the Author

Born into a family tragically impacted by type 1 diabetes (T1D), and living with a sister and a son with T1D, Bonnie O'Neil has a keen understanding of the impact of chronic illness on a family. She has channeled her insight into her work as an advocate for funding for T1D research and education.

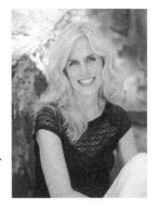

Bonnie serves as a board member of the founding chapter of JDRF, the Juvenile Diabetes Research Foundation—the leading global organization funding T1D research. She has served the board in many capacities, including board president, and she speaks regularly at JDRF education conferences and events.

Bonnie is a spiritual director and the executive director of Alpha Mid Atlantic, a faith-based nonprofit. She formerly worked as a banker in New York and Boston before moving to Paris, where she earned her MA in French.

Bonnie has made her home in several other East Coast towns and lived for two years in London. She now lives in suburban Philadelphia with her husband, Jon. Together they look forward to every opportunity to spend time with their three adult children, Alexander, Austin, and Alicia.

You can keep up with Bonnie at bonnieoneil.com and on Instagram and Facebook.